HYPNOSIS AND FALSE MEMORIES
How False Memories Are Created

By Ronald L. Stephens, Msc.D., C.Ht.

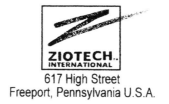

ZIOTECH..
INTERNATIONAL
617 High Street
Freeport, Pennsylvania U.S.A.

HYPNOSIS AND FALSE MEMORIES
How False Memories Are Created

By Ronald L. Stephens, Msc.D., C.Ht.

Edited by Joyce Davis

Published by:

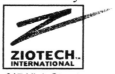

ZIOTECH International
617 High Street
Freeport, Pennsylvania U.S.A.

Copyright © 1995, 1996
First Printing 1996
Printed in the United States of America

Library of Congress Catalog Card Number: 95-90201
Stephens, Ronald L.
HYPNOSIS AND FALSE MEMORIES: How False Memories are Created
Bibliography: p.
Includes index.
1. Hypnosis - Handbooks, manuals, etc. I. Title
2. False Memories - Psychology
3. Psychology - Handbooks, manuals, etc.
4. Law Enforcement - Handbooks, manuals, etc.
5. Law - Handbooks, manuals, etc.
616.858
ISBN 0-9646392-0-3: $12.95 Softcover

Table of Contents

FOREWORD

There we were, all 270 passengers, loaded on the plane and ready to take off for our destination. Some were going to work, some were going to play while others were to returning home. Wherever each of us was going, we were ready. Our bags were on the plane, our seat belts fastened, and suddenly a voice came over the speaker system. "We regret to inform you of a slight delay, we forgot to check to see if the crew had arrived and unfortunately, we have no pilot."

How many therapists are ready to go only to find out they don't have a pilot? Well, go ahead and pack your bags, our pilot has arrived. Dr. Ronald Stephens has given us a much needed flight plan. As I read this book, I wondered if inadvertently I had "triggered false memories." As you read this book, you will find yourself examining your own practices as a therapist. You will soon ask yourself: Am I using leading phrases or are my inductions proper? Do I understand the power of the words I use? Am I really listening to clients or am I assuming that I know what they mean? What kind of legal trouble could I be in and what kind of heartache might I cause for families?

From the moment you start to read this book you will begin to look at your own practices. This book contains a wealth of information that we all need to have. Thanks' Ron. You have given us so much important information and it makes us think about what we are doing.

Barbara L. Coman, Ph.D.
President, Coman & Associates
Los Angeles, California

PREFACE

Therapists know that hypnosis will reduce a person's resistance of bringing repressed memories to the surface. The process, however, is not without limitations. If the client is led during the session, the therapist has increased the possibilities that the memories may be false. Therapists should be aware of their role and responsibilities during hypnosis to recover a client's memories. They should understand that their actions may contribute to altering the accuracy of those memories. It is the therapist's responsibility to insure against creating false memories. This book will provide basic information in preventing that from occurring.

ACKNOWLEDGMENTS

I would like to express my deepest gratitude to the many clients, organizations and fellow therapists with whom I have worked throughout the years. The ideas presented in this book belong to each of you and provided the necessary foundation needed to complete the task. I would like to thank my family and friends for their support and patience during the endless hours of research and writing. I would also like to thank Joyce Davis, whom I consider to be a master editor, for her inexhaustible efforts. It was her willingness to accept the draft manuscript and turn it into comprehensible writing that finally made the effort worthwhile. Thanks to each of you for playing such an important part of my life. May heaven's bright lights shine on each of you, forever.

DISCLAIMER

The intention of this book is to provide information regarding the subject matter covered. Ziotech International is selling this publication with the understanding that the publisher and author are not engaged in rendering legal or other professional services. If you do require legal assistance or other expert advice, you should seek the services of a competent professional.

It is not the purpose of this book to reprint all the information that is otherwise available to the author and/or publisher, but to complement other texts. For more information, see the bibliography listing at the end of this publication or contact those entities mentioned in the text.

We have attempted to make this manual as complete and as accurate as possible. However, it is possible that mistakes, both typographical and in content, may exist. Therefore, you should use this text only as a general guide and not as the ultimate source of hypnosis and false memory information. Furthermore, this book contains information on the subject only up to the printing date.

The purpose of this book is awareness. The author and Ziotech International shall have neither liability nor responsibility to any person or entity with respect to any loss or damage caused, or alleged to be caused, directly or indirectly by the information contained in this book.

If you do not wish to be bound by the above, you may return this book to the publisher for a full refund.

"We're all on a journey, and some of us know it, and some don't."

Steven Seagal

CHAPTER ONE

THE JOURNEY

Through the years, many books have been written on the subject of false memories. Few addressed what was really happening regarding the accuracy of memories recalled while an individual was in a state of hypnosis. A few authors investigated the role of therapists concerning false memories. Fewer still addressed the possibility that therapists were "leading" their client while the subject was in a high state of suggestibility. Of those few, the authors appeared to ignore the importance of words and wording in surfacing memories that are totally false. Until now, the connection between hypnosis, the therapist, and false memories appeared insignificant. This book is a journey to correct that void and to prevent future errors from surfacing. This is a journey toward the suppression of false memories.

FALSE MEMORIES

What does the successful therapist know about false memories that an unsuccessful therapist does not? Most would base a therapist's success on his knowledge of human behavior, stages of man's development, application of therapeutic techniques and professional mannerisms. They would not exclude his entrepreneur dynamics coupled with an understanding of private practice, civil law and his insatiable deep passion to know more. Those who are unsuccessful *think* they know enough. They usually spend their time defending what little they do know, instead of discovering what they don't know.

Successful therapists have determination to get it right. They are compulsive about detail. They focus their attention on the multitude of seemingly insignificant and unimportant words that make up their daily scripts. The words and the script, when executed correctly, become the distinctive essence that distinguishes the superlative from the mediocre.

Successful therapists realize they have an impact on memories. Those therapists realize that they are part of a process that can create false memories, by words, actions, or premise.

In a national publication, the headline reads, "A Father Fights Back." The headline drew national attention. Recalled memory of a daughter's childhood sexual molestation by her father became important to the news media. It became even more important when the case centered on false memories, possibly triggered by a therapist's line of questioning. The father aimed his suit at the therapist. The courtroom battle not only interested the public, but therapists across the nation watched with poignant interest. Anyone associated with any aspect of therapy had concerns. The result of this case could affect livelihoods. Lawyers placed legitimate sexual abuse cases uncovered in regressive therapy on hold. They were reluctant to take on a case that involved regressive therapy. The abused were reluctant to move forward in fear of retaliation or ridicule. What followed was even more shocking.

Headlines of the nation's newspapers barked, "Father Accused of Incest Wins Suit Against Memory Therapist!" A California jury awarded him a half million dollars.

This case was more than it appeared to all concerned. It awakened therapists to the possibility of lawsuits. They now knew that what they said and how they said it was important. Therapists knew they could no longer base anything on a premise. They also understood that they could trigger false memories by a single word. They knew, for instance, they shouldn't be insistent that certain eating disorders were necessarily the result of childhood sexual abuse. They knew that they might have to prove their findings. Liability insurance for therapists began to climb.

Across the nation, books emerged on the subject of false memories. Organizations initiated studies to uncover inappropriate techniques and methods. Therapists from Seattle to Sarasota divided into their perspective camps. Some groups were protective of their techniques and methods while others were seeing the need for change. Questions arose. Who is liable for triggering false memories? Do states have laws relating to these cases? California does! In California, therapists are liable for their actions and are subject to lawsuits. Other states have begun to develop similar laws to protect the public.

Investigations arose in the use of sodium amytal

treatment. Most know it by its common name of truth serum. The public slowly became aware, as did many therapists, that patients treated with sodium amytal are also responsive to suggestion. On that basis alone, it is not admissible in court.

Where does the therapist turn? We can never know what memories are 100 percent true. Nevertheless, a point does exist at which therapists need to believe in the veracity of their patient's memories - in any event, at least acknowledging that the patients themselves believe them to be true.

Therapists must be aware, however, that a distorted memory process does exist, that a client's memory recall may be delusional in some way, even psychotic. Perhaps the individual is trying to get attention. It cannot be overlooked that to the patient the experience is real. Therapists must always have some doubts during the process and constantly evaluate their patient. The evaluation must have a starting point. Initially, addressing the memory as if it is real may provide a beginning. The distorted memory will surface during hypnosis. To some, the uncovering of a distorted memory may seem difficult. If a therapist has doubts in his own training, knowledge or techniques, and if his ego allows him, he should refer the client to someone better qualified.

For many years, a belief that eating disorders stemmed from childhood sexual abuse was common. Today, the breach in the link between eating disorders and sexual disorders is widening. A recent study at the Harvard Medical School, published in the American Journal of Psychiatry (April 1992), concluded that there is no support for the idea that sexual abuse is a great risk factor for bulimia.

When some therapists collect data from their clients and state that they believe they can trace eating disorders to about 80% of the sexual abuse cases, they are offering what we call "process suggestion." It is still suggestion. Some therapists will continue their witch hunt although the client has recovered very accurate memories to the contrary.

A therapist must accept the idea that the client has to find a reason for his problem. The client usually has exposed himself to all the self-help books, talk shows, magazine articles, etc., on moving forward with his life. He now has the notion that he will never move forward unless he knows where his internal conflicts originated. Until he accomplishes this, he thinks he will never be normal. Often, when he is in therapy, the client feels safer. Finally, someone will listen. Trying to uncover some unsettling information from the past, he will rely on the therapist to guide him. Some therapists will do just that, and guide the client by suggestion. The suggestions may be direct, indirect, processed or unprocessed. Removing all suggestion from this setting is impossible.

No basis exists for disbelieving or invalidating someone's memory. There is no rationale for questioning what a client may be experiencing. The concern begins when somebody walks in to a therapists office, and describes himself as "depressed, anxious, and having poor self-esteem." There is even more cause for concern when the therapist, basing his evaluation on a premise, says, "Well, I know what that is all about.".

Some therapists continue the premise by describing possible childhood events, repressed memories, and denial. Continuing this course of action is common for some therapists, even though the client has said, "Well, I don't have any memories like that!" Some therapists will slowly convince the person that they do, indeed, have memories, and that these are true memories, and they give substance to his anxiety. In this setting these clinicians are not really doing their job. They are making an interpretation without first asking the patient what he thinks the underlying causes of his problems might be. The therapist is not a mind reader.

Many books written on the subject of memory explain that confrontation is part of the therapy. Therapists have recently interpreted confrontation to include public disclosure and lawsuits. They feel they have to bring this forward, make it public, and then make the guilty party pay for his crimes. This is all under the guise of therapy. Therapy is not litigation. Therapy should bring families together and work through difficulties.

The following is an excerpt from an actual case in which the young lady withdrew her charges against her father. Efforts were successful to reunite the family.

"So I went to work on trauma searching, and ended up, four years later, worse off than I went in. It was like having a nightmare, only I was awake. At one point, he would hypnotize me or put me to sleep or count down or whatever to relax, but I had a hard time. I struggled with them. He insisted that they were true, and I had to find those memories."

In another well-publicized case in 1990, a daughter's accusation of murder against her father shocked a nation. This case, Eileen Franklin verses George Franklin, became a trend setter. This trial provided the legal precedence and ground work needed for therapists and lawyers to surface other cases. This case involved the murder of nine-year-old Susan Kay Nason on December 2, 1969, twenty miles Southwest of San Francisco. During the murder trial, Eileen Franklin revealed how memories began to surface twenty years later. Her recall began as flashbacks while watching one of her own children lying on the floor. Confused about the images, she chose to enter therapy to better understand the recurring events. During therapy, Ms. Franklin recalled memories of seeing her father bludgeon her childhood playmate twenty years earlier. She spoke of Susan trying to shield herself from the blows and testified that one of the blows crushed the ring she was wearing on her left hand. True or false, the accusations were enough to sentence her father to life in prison. Besides the father's sentencing, the real tragedy of this particular case was the quotation by Eileen's therapist. Court documents revealed the therapist's blasé attitude concerning her therapy and strong accusations. He said, "My purpose really was just to help her have those memories. I told her it wasn't important whether they were real or not."

We all should be rallying against this kind of procedure. Nobody should have to confront these types of suggestions and attitudes. Richard Ofshe, the author of *Making Monsters*, which addresses false memories and their impact on society carries the same concerns. When interviewed by a television reporter on the subject of false memories, he said these people are being "victimized by their therapists. They were told by supposedly well trained, competent, experts on this, their therapists, that these visualizations are real."

For a moment, place yourself in the shoes of the client. How would you feel after months of agony, only to discover that your memory was a lie, and you were the victim of inappropriate therapy?

Every situation is different. When we look at the broad spectrum of these cases, we know that some therapists will jump to conclusions. It is their only way to explain what is happening to the client. Some therapists keep pressuring the client, believing they are in denial, that they may be repressing memory.

When we look in any childhood, we will always find children who do repress memories for whatever reason. Memories of one's childhood take on a faded quality, distorted and softened around the edges by the ever widening distance between the present and the past. We all forget some memories, especially if they were traumatic. That is a miracle of the mind. When something is so horrible that we want to block it out, the mind obliges. Later, in an effort to recall those horrendous events, therapists must help individuals sort through the rubbish to find the truth. Is it possible to accomplish this without leading the individual? It is, but it is a monumental task.

Today, the task has risks. Clients can sue therapists and hold them accountable. It is a sad commentary, especially at this period in our culture when families most need communication. It is as though therapists are splintering clients and families saying, "You don't need to talk."

Therapists need to know how to diagnose without jumping to conclusions when there is insufficient evidence. The clients are searching hard for answers to their questions, and some therapists will oblige.

From a legal stand, proving repressed memories in court is tough. Disproving them is even tougher. We must always remember some flashbacks are very real, just not reality.

FALSE MEMORY SYNDROME

This new phenomenon has not only separated families, it has jammed the court rooms, employed hundreds of lawyers, and has been seen on nearly all of television's daytime talk shows. It is constantly in the public's eye, and on their mind. Well-known Hollywood celebrities have jumped on the bandwagon to hide behind the cloak of abuse, based on false memories.

Recalling memories of childhood sexual abuse, satanic cult abuse, etc., has become the "in" thing, the fad of the nineties. Many of these memories are false. We all have inaccurate, or layered, memories stored in our mind's recall section. Has the fascination for recovered memories reached its apex? It hasn't if the entertainment media continues to play to its homage. Authors have written hundreds of books on the subject and these will continue to be best sellers until the circumstances change. What is going on here?

Dr. John F. Kihlstrom, Ph.D., best defined False Memory Syndrome (FMS) as, "a condition in which a person's identity and interpersonal relationships are centered around a memory of traumatic experience which is objectively false but in which the person strongly believes. Note that the syndrome is not characterized by false memories as such. We all have memories that are inaccurate. Rather, the syndrome may be diagnosed when the memory is so deeply ingrained that it orients the individual's entire personality and lifestyle, in turn disrupting all sorts of other adaptive behavior. The analogy to personality disorder is intentional. False Memory Syndrome is especially destructive because the person assiduously avoids confrontation with any evidence that might challenge the memory. Thus it takes on a life of its own, encapsulated and resistant to correction. The person may become so focused on memory that he or she may be effectively distracted from coping with the real problems in his or her life."

In March 1992, affected families and some of the nation's top professionals joined forces to establish the False Memory Syndrome Foundation (FMSF). The Foundation, based in Philadelphia, Pennsylvania, established several goals. They wanted to provide a clearing house for this new phenomenon that was sweeping the nation. The Foundation set out to study the origins, distribute the latest scientific information on memory to the public and professional community, and in return to provide help to affected families.

Immediately, when people hear of such a Foundation they fear that it will cause a backlash and the public will believe that sexual abuse of children doesn't exist. The Foundation is attempting to see that no backlash occurs. They, like everyone else, believe that sexual abuse of children is a reprehensible crime. Their efforts are not to thwart the exposure of sexual child abuse, but to ensure that we substantiate all evidence and that therapists scrutinize memory enhancement techniques to prevent the creation of false memories.

EVERYONE HAS A ROLE IN THE PROCESS

Memory researchers believe that anytime we recall an event and discuss it in detail, we are creating new images for storage (See Section II on Layering). This means that a casual conversation of the "good old days" is *layering* different images for us to recall later. Anytime we ask leading questions about certain details when someone is recalling an event, we have become part of the process. It doesn't matter whether that event took place an hour, days, or even years ago.

We each face the possibility of triggering false memories whether we want to or not. When, for example, a sexual violation of a little girl occurs, several individuals become entangled in the network of support. Most try to be sensitive during this despicable tragedy and they offer support as they know it. Most do not really comprehend what involvement is taking place. Follow along for just a moment as we explore how several individuals, without realizing their involvement, often "lead" and "create" memories.

Even at the age of eight years old, Becky knows what has taken place is wrong. She has a difficult time. Should she tell someone or keep it to herself? She wants to tell her mother, yet she doesn't want her mother to think badly of her. She finally builds up enough courage to confide in her mother. From this moment, the formation of false memories may begin.

Trying to be a good parent, the mother may ask some simple questions to comfort Becky. Both are still in a state of total confusion. The little girl, trying to satisfy her mother, stumbles over words. The mother, out of deep compassion for the hurt and embarrassment of her daughter, offers assistance - - a couple of words to best describe the incident. The original scene is undergoing some cleansing and a new image is beginning to take shape. In the child's memory bank, she is "layering" these new images over the original scene.

The mother, angry and hurt, and rightfully so, wants the violator brought to justice. She notifies the police. Once contacted, the police notify Social Services and send an investigator to analyze the situation.

Becky is now experiencing even more embarrassment. Not only was it difficult trying to tell her mother, but now she has to tell a complete stranger. Becky's "private self" is experiencing an invasion. She also wants to satisfy her mother by doing everything right. When she stumbles in re-telling the event, the investigator and her mother continue to offer their thoughts, their words. She agrees. Poor Becky, the original scene has undergone a second coat of paint. New sets of images are layered into her memory bank.

The investigator, satisfied with the information, notifies the police who take appropriate criminal action. Meanwhile, Becky's mother is aware of her daughter's emotional condition and calls her minister. Again, Becky must open her soul to the world and repeat the details of the incident.

No researcher can guarantee that the original scene, as recalled by Becky, is accurate. It may be a composite of the three previous confessions, using words and descriptions offered by her mother, the investigator and the minister.

The minister usually asks questions to decide if Becky may need therapy. Embarrassment is now becoming a constant. In her shyness, Becky may have held back some details or descriptions. Realizing what has taken place, the minister recommends a therapist.

Becky experiences devastation, hurt, anger, guilt and sadness. She must again relay the story to the therapist, where her mother may not be present. Will the therapist, if he does not fully understand layering, add to the scene? Will Becky be able to recall the original incident? Or, will her story finally be a composite as her mother, the investigator, the minister and her therapist described the event? No one can be sure. Whatever account she describes, will she layer it also with the original? How accurately will it portray what actually occurred?

Finally, we reach the grand finale of little Becky's frightful experience. Criminal charges against the violator will not take place until Becky makes a deposition of the incident to a court reporter.

What she conveys to the court reporter may be exactly as Becky recalls of the original scene, or it may be a composite of several layers of images. By now, chances are her story is a composite of many viewpoints. It is not Becky's fault. This scenario belongs to each of us. Parents have not received training in proper techniques of questioning. Most people do not know exactly what "leading questions" are. Often, Social Service workers, police, religious leaders, and most therapists do not know.

Is there a solution to this situation? Public awareness may be the only answer. Some metropolitan police forces and women's organizations are attempting to educate the public. They emphasize the importance of giving a deposition as close to the event as possible. Some of them understand "leading" and "layering." They may use other terms, but it all means the same thing: TRUTH may have become half-truth, or outright fiction.

"Wisdom ofttimes consists of knowing what to do next."
-Herbert Hoover

> "Open minds, like open windows,
> need screens to keep
> the bugs out."
>
> Richard K. Rudolph

CHAPTER TWO

WHAT DO WE REALLY KNOW ABOUT MEMORY?

Memory is difficult to measure. However, researchers have made great strides trying to understand the essence of memory. The process is slow. Memory research has not experienced the great leaps and bounds of the computer chip. Nothing is as complex as the inner workings of the mind. Most of the inner workings of memory remain a mystery.

After years of research, it appears that the more we've learned about memory, the less we know. It may take another two-thousand-years to fully understand the sum and substance of memory.

Researchers have confirmed the existence of areas

within the brain that appear to correspond with recollection of memory. This information on memory recall is important to our false memory research. It has also been discovered that memory is a stimulated release of sensations, sounds, sights, and smells. Researchers agree that in a conscious state, memories involving names, faces, images, dates, or situations are more difficult to recall than physical motor memories. The physical motor memories are those functions we stored when we learned to ride a bicycle, play golf, swim or bowl. It involves the combination and coordination of every muscle and action of the body.

Memory researchers generally agree on some things. They believe we can separate memory into two main facets, short term memory and long term memory. Short term memory (STM) is information that we only retain for a few moments, thirty seconds or so, unless we attempt to keep it longer. They often call STM our "working memory." It processes and stores information for as long as we actively think about it. Long term memory (LTM), on the other hand, involves memory that has exceeded the STM temporary information bank and becomes stored permanently somewhere in the confines of the mind. Exactly what is LTM? Researchers now realize that LTM is storage of an event that got our full attention when it occurred. Researchers now understand that event has to be something novel, wonderful, repetitive, emotionally intense, noisy, horrifying or of special interest to cause the individual to focus on it so intently.

Some believe we retain our original LTM forever. Surfacing the information in a conscious state may be difficult for some. Each of us has had the experience of trying in vain to recall the name of that special young classmate who once escorted us to the prom, or the date of Aunt Josie's birthday, or where we put the car insurance papers. Sometimes we worry that we may be losing our minds. Specific reasons for our inability to recall memories at specific moments have come to light. Sometimes we clutter recollection of details, while in a conscious state, with the conditions surrounding us at a specific moment. Nullifying those conditions with the use of hypnosis is possible. Once nullified, the process of recall can begin without clutter. LTM is an area of concern among individuals trained in the use of hypnosis, because it also encases the possibility of false memories.

FEELINGS AND MEMORIES

Emotions affect the ability to recall. Study upon study reveals additional understanding of memories and their impact on our lives. The memory of a past experience and recalling how it made us feel, when it occurred, can be as powerfully arousing as the original event itself. An individual can heighten or lessen the intensity of those feelings. The intensity comes from how we think and what we remember. Retrieval cues can enhance intensity.

We should understand the meanings of several terms before we continue any further. To some they seem interchangeable, however they are different and distinct. The words are **recognition** and **recall**. **Recognition** is the ability to **identify** something that the individual has previously encountered, or been exposed to. It does not matter whether the information is old, new, correct or incorrect. **Recall** is the ability to **retrieve and reproduce** information that is not currently present. Recall is more difficult to accomplish than recognition.

Recognition occurs when a witness to a crime recognizes an individual from police files or in a line up. The mind processes recognition differently. It sorts through an endless list of facial features and compares each of them until it matches the one remembered.

Recall, on the other hand, is the ability to retrieve endless details of a person, place, thing or an event. During recall, individuals surface detail that involves color, smell, emotions, touch, shapes, sounds, scenes, dates, numbers, objects, and the behaviors and actions of people.

During the process of recall, another phenomenon has entered the picture and to some extent its use has been successful. They call these phenomenon "retrieval cues." Retrieval cues are markers present at the time of the initial experience. Retrieval is often easier when the individual is in the same physical and emotional state as when he stored the information originally. Physically, a client may take the fetal position during recall as the scene begins to unfold. It may even be a whiff of his mother's sweet perfume, a dog barking, or the taste of mother's warm home-made bread that can recall a specific memory.

A few therapists are using retrieval cues successfully. However, one must take extreme precautions that the cue is not leading the individual. Authorities consider it leading if the therapist shows a witness a disturbing photograph of a murder scene before the recall induction, just to get her into the same emotional and physical state. If they were to show the her a photograph of the suspect and they have already proved, beyond any doubt, that the suspect was at the scene, it may not be leading. Weighing all aspects of the situation before proceeding with retrieval cues is wise. Remember, it may not be the therapist's responsibility to judge. In a legal case, the attorneys may have to decide if the retrieval cues are leading.

Researchers have uncovered some interesting facts concerning violent crimes and recall. It has been discovered that victims of violent crimes often have trouble recalling details of their experience. It appears the difficulties surface because they are not at the same level of emotional arousal that they were at the time of the crime. The research does not mean, however, that people must be emotionally aroused to the original level to recall the violence.

Studies reveal a significant breakthrough in aspects of recall in depressed individuals. The mind of a depressed person often surfaces unhappy memories. That is why the pre-induction interview between a client and therapist is extremely important. The emotional condition of the individual will usually surface during this first meeting. In addition, and equally important, the therapist may unconsciously enhance the client's unhappiness by leading words, such as, "You must have been extremely upset when you received word of her death." Couple that statement with sad background music and you have directed her toward utter gloom.

MEMORY AND PASSAGE OF TIME

Most experts on memory believe that some details drop out of our memory, *in a conscious state*, with the passage of time. They predict that, within a year of the event, individuals in a conscious state trying to recall an event may have lost about 20 percent. After five years, it is estimated that we lose as high as 60 percent of the details. They conducted the measurements in a normally awakened state. They also understand that under hypnosis, a person can recall details normally considered lost in an awakened or conscious state.

Stages of recall during hypnosis may be "cue dependent." The individual may alter his own physical or emotional state by "revisiting" the event and recover long forgotten details that he once thought were lost. Many of us have had noteworthy experiences of clients "revisiting" a traumatic event in their life. Trained therapists are aware of how to handle these *revisits.*

Allow me to share some insight on revisits. During regression, the individual's revisit of a trauma can occur unexpectedly. What occurs during that revisit can also be frightful for anyone witnessing the client's encounter with those scenes. That includes the therapist. During one such occurrence, a tiny 47-year-old migrant woman was recalling her rape by a brother-in-law when she was thirteen. The event took place the very afternoon that she arrived in the United States from Mexico. Speaking very little English and knowing no one, this small childlike creature accepted her sister's hospitality. Her acceptance later proved disastrous.

The woman's husband had requested to sit in during the session. As she reached a particular point of recalling the event she huddled on the recliner in a fetal position. Her legs curled up tightly against her body while her arms seemingly were pushing away her unwanted attacker. The woman's entire body quivered and she began to sob vehemently. The absence of the attacker made no difference. In her mind, the attack was fresh and real. During the revisit she had recalled the minute details. Her caring husband rushed to her side, wanting to comfort her. Fortunately for me, he was a frail little man who proved non threatening and I could restrain him from interrupting her *revisit.*

The pros and cons of allowing or not allowing the

client to go through a revisit trauma is a personal matter. It should be the call of the client and therapist. The *joint* decision hinges on the precise needs of the client to remember details. My client, her husband, and I had discussed her needs in great detail. Her present sexual apprehensions, failure to enjoy sexual intercourse, her disgust for the male form and verification of the attacker had to surface from this recall and *revisit*. Trained therapists can assist in the recollection of details during a revisit without leading the individual.

LONG TERM MEMORIES (LTM)

To understand LTM, we need to understand what kinds of memories the brain can store. Memories are categorized into three general types: procedural, semantic, and episodic.

A procedural memory surfaces a particular action, such as how to brush your teeth or drive a car. Semantic memories include facts, rules, and concepts - - you have to be out of the hotel room by 10 AM. -- the capital of California is Sacramento. Episodic memories are personally experienced events, the memories of the past - - that flat tire in Indianapolis, your first kiss. Today, memory experts have even linked semantic and episodic memories together as "declarative memories." The declarative memories are those we will concentrate on for recall.

Many memory studies have revealed that when we consciously recall information, we actually remember some and reconstruct the rest. Often we cannot tell what we originally stored and what we have added since the event. It all feels like one memory (See Layering). The bits and pieces, from accumulated sources, would be hard to define.

Today, continuing research has revealed that we not only reconstruct memories at the time of recall, but we alter information even as we are storing it. We alter the information into categories to make the recall process simpler. We will store the information that we decide to be important to us in LTM. Any participant in a memory recall research program is really determining, at a given moment, if what he is storing is important to him. We have no way of knowing what is important to that individual. We have no way of knowing what the individual process is for determining what is important enough to store in the LTM bank. This type of research, referred to as *controlled research*, seems almost useless. Individuals participating in this type of memory research program are told that details they are about to hear are important. They are also reminded to remember the details. It is difficult, if not completely impossible, to tell someone what they should store or not store in long term memory. The next thousand years may not reveal exactly what evaluation process is taking place within the confines of the mind to select what information we want to store in LTM.

THE RETRIEVAL PROCESS

Many psychologists and researchers have concluded that retrieval is the key process in remembering and forgetting. Forgetting information usually involves external interference. New memories, or layering, interferes with old memories. Another theory is that we often forget simply because we want to forget, or because it was not important to us at the time. The use of hypnosis for recall is a powerful tool. Often, an individual can recall old memories when he becomes oblivious to his present surroundings. In addition, under hypnosis most people are capable of intense concentration on whatever is suggested to them. However, any indication of leading the individual in a state of hypnosis can alter recall.

"Under hypnosis, the natural tendency to confuse fact and speculation is increased both by a desire to please the hypnotist and by the fact that hypnosis encourages fantasy and vivid imagery."

Wade & Tavris

Recall, or retrieval, is a reconstructive process. We should note that most people who reconstruct the past are not deliberately lying. They recall what they can reconstruct. If someone gave them a polygraph test during a hypnosis recall session, where no leading has taken place, they would probably pass.

Our memory can play tricks. In a conscious state we often remember things that never happened and forget things that did take place. Even recent memories can evaporate as quickly as spilled rubbing alcohol. However, regressive memory can also be remarkably accurate. We each retain in memory hundreds of thousands of facts, descriptions, and skills, available to us in an instant if revisited properly.

Jean Piaget, a Swiss psychologist, once wrote a paper of his earliest memories. In his writing he recalled a near kidnapping at the age of two. His recollection of the details surrounding the event appeared flawless. Piaget impressed those close to him with his story. He recalled sitting in a baby carriage, watching his nurse defend him from the would-be kidnappers. Piaget added minor details when he told of the scratches she received on her face. He strengthened his story when he described a police officer with a cloak and white baton, and remembered the officer chasing the kidnappers away.

The story of Piaget's detailed recollection never happened. When he was fifteen, his parents received a letter from his former nurse confessing that she had made up the entire story. Piaget later wrote of his recalled memory, "I therefore must have heard, as a child, the account of this story . . . and projected it into the past in the form of a visual memory, which was a memory of a memory, but false."

"When I was younger I could remember anything, whether it happened or not."

Mark Twain

Each of us is, in a real sense, the sum of personal recollections. We used to think of memory as similar to that of an imprint in hot waxes, and any imprints left there are there forever. Some have even called our memory a tape recorder, saying that it records every moment of our lives. These perceptions are misleading. If they were true, our minds would experience unnecessary clutter and a fill of insignificant mental garbage. In actuality, our memory is highly selective.

What gets stored in memory is not a replica of the experience. For example, we change sensory information in form almost as soon as we detect it, and the form retained for a long term is different from the original stimulation. When we hear the President of the United States at a press conference, we do not store every word verbatim. Instead, we convert sentences to units of meaning made up of abstract concepts rather than words. We encode those concepts in some fashion for later retrieval. We can store information in other forms similar to visual or auditory images. Visual memories are often more accurate. Other forms, such as those that allow us to ride a bicycle, we store as muscular instructions. Professional athletes store muscular instructions so they can repeat the motions with great precision.

SUPPRESSED MEMORIES

The human mind is fascinating. Researchers have unveiled volumes of material designed to explain and to understand the mind and how it works. They know that the mind, to protect us from discomfort, harm, pain and tragic events, will suppress those memories that trigger remembrance of such events. They call them repressed memories. Repressed memories are a specific group normally excluded from our conscious state. An individual can recall those events, using hypnosis and guided imagery. The research also revealed that leading questions can trigger a false image of those events. Today, the acceptable term associated with these memories and this type of therapy is Recovered Memory Therapy (RMT).

A client in his search for truth may want to uncover the details of a suppressed memory. The therapist has an obligation to see that the client's recall belongs totally to the client. He has an obligation to word his questions carefully so the client may describe events and totally recall in great detail without any interference.

During the surfacing of a repressed memory, the client may experience some discomfort and pain. A caring therapist often wants to help the patient. The words "therapist" and "caretaker" are synonymous. However, in assisting, the therapist can also destroy or alter the recall. The assistance may seem insignificant, like finishing a difficult sentence for them. Possibly it could even be providing a particular word to describe a specific scene. It all seems like such a little task that appears harmless. But once the therapist interjects his or her own thoughts by projecting a description, color, size, shape or situation during the effort to recall, they are misleading the client. The therapist has begun to trigger a false memory.

Getting back on track is virtually impossible. With the interjection of one word, we taint the scene. Under hypnosis, usually considered the best possible method of retrieving uncontaminated memories, we have changed the picture. No one will ever know what is real.

Subsequent sessions to address the same situation may not be flawless either, since the mind continues to develop new images. By the interjection of a single word during a suppressed or repressed memory recall session, the therapist may have created a new image. With a stroke of the brush the artist can ruin a magnificent painting.

RECALL

To understand fully how we can create false memories, we should understand the process known as "recall". Recall, as it applies to the mind, is simply "an act of remembering a person, place, thing, event or experience." Notice that the definition does not allude to a hypnotic state. Recall is a process of the mind to reintroduce us to something that we have stored in our memory bank, consciously, or subconsciously.

In actuality, we experience this "state of call back" constantly throughout each day. Anytime we reminisce about old times with family and friends we are in a state of recall.

We are reviving old memories.

A direct connection exists between recall and our state of consciousness. There are three levels of consciousness: the conscious, the preconscious (or fore conscious), and the subconscious. Each state of consciousness functions and recalls different subjects. For example, the conscious state is that level of mental awareness in direct contact with reality. The preconscious exists between the conscious and the subconscious. During the preconscious state we recall such things as data, concepts, and experiences readily. However, the recalled information rarely has any association with emotional conflicts or deeper drives. We usually think of it as ordinary memory association. The subconscious is the repository for repressed emotional experiences and bypasses subject awareness.

A regressive hypnosis session may fluctuate between the preconscious and the subconscious. The electroencephalogram (EEG) tests that have determined six recordable levels of hypnosis encompass that spectrum between the preconscious and the subconscious. Hypnosis heightens the responsiveness during recall in both states.

A most notable and recorded case of recall occurred in 1976, near Chowchilla, California. One hot summer afternoon, someone driving a van forced a bus carrying a load of school children off the road. Boarding the bus, the kidnappers forced the driver and children to exit and transported them to a stone quarry. There, they locked everyone inside a large trailer. A taupe, covered with dirt and debris, camouflaged the trailer from anyone searching from the air. They planned to hold their hostages for ransom.

Later, the bus driver managed to remove a riveted air vent from the roof of the trailer. He hoisted several small children through the tiny opening and they ran for help.

Fortunately, the rest of the children and the bus driver were rescued from the hot summer sun. However, no one could describe the van that forced them off the road.

Under hypnosis, the bus driver could recall all but one of the license plate numbers on the kidnapper's van. He subconsciously recorded the license plate numbers that flashed before his eyes as he was forced off the road. He gave two numbers, a three and an eight, as possibilities for an unclear number. His recall provided enough information for the authorities to arrest and eventually convict the kidnappers.

Believing that the driver couldn't possibly recall all of the numbers, the therapist went to check the kidnapper's van which the police had impounded. Rust and dirt had partially obliterated the number the bus driver had difficulty recalling, so he could not see it clearly. It was an eight.

The driver proved again that, under hypnosis, we can recall information many researchers believe is unavailable. What can interfere with recall? We have narrowed possible interference from three sources: drugs (prescription, non-prescription, and illegal), extremely poor circulation, or trauma that caused damages directly to the brain. A fourth category has surfaced - - the bungled efforts of an inexperienced practitioner unfamiliar with proper hypnotic techniques.

LAYERING

Understanding the process of "layering" is important to understanding false memories fully. Layering is often defined as a process of simply laying new images over old images. Most researchers believe once layering has occurred, the chance of recalling the original image becomes infinitesimal without hypnosis. Once layering has occurred, any recalled images may become a composite of the old and the newly added images.

When does the actual process of layering occur? Nobody knows. It is an unknown in memory research. Some believe that anytime we recall any image, during any process, make any changes or alterations implied or imagined to the original scene, we layer the new images among the old images. This process can even take place in the awakened state. Individuals who have heard a story repeatedly from someone they trust or admire may eventually begin to believe the event took place. The belief system is strong. Couple the belief system with new descriptions or added details and the individual creates another scene, layered on the original.

Since childhood we have been told the story of the crucifixion of Jesus. Using a lie-detector and asked properly, we would verify that the event took place although we never witnessed it. Most individuals carry countless stories their parents repeated throughout their childhood. Many of the events never happened. However, the parents believed the stories to be true because their own parents told them, whether it is the story of their great-grandfather's heroic efforts during the Civil War, or their great aunt's discovery of pancakes. Each time the story is told it is embellished with added details. The embellishment makes it more believable. As children we processes these stories as truth. Our parents wouldn't lie to us, so it must be true. Every child will verbalize those same stories for years until the images become ingrained in their memory bank.

Later, during a state of regression for example, if it is suggested that certain events are taking place, we may store the new image with the original. Let us digress a moment to fully understand the concept. Suppose that you are trying to recall an event and the image surfaces as you remember it: a woman is standing on a small bridge overlooking a peaceful river. Her name is Mary and she is a close friend of yours. She is trying to steady herself. She holds onto the railing of the bridge with one hand. She wears a long red coat. As you recall the scene, you are behind her and she is looking away from you.

If, during a recall session, or even in a conscious state during a casual discussion with a friend, you recall a scene and make any changes to your original scene, you will store it as a version of the original. If you recall the scene in a conscious state, and during your conversation with someone, they interject that Mary did not own a red coat, our layering has started to take form. However, they said, she did have a long lavender coat. You will create and store a new scene with the original scene by layering. Later, the image may surface with Mary wearing a lavender coat. It does not seem to matter what process you are using to recall that moment. Also, it may surface with her wearing a red coat, but she does not have her hand on the bridge railing because someone else suggested that particular bridge did not have a railing. Later, a therapist in another recall session asks if she wore a hat and shoes, and was it a river or a stream? The insertions of new words constantly create new images layered upon the original scene.

The human mind is constantly in a state of gathering, updating, storing and recalling information. Innocent as any conversation may seem, the mind is creative and paints new pictures. That process is forever ongoing. As therapists, we must be certain that we are not adding to the process by inserting information during a hypnosis recall session. The insertion of suggestions in this type of therapy is unwarranted. The individual is highly susceptible to suggestion. Dr. William S. Kroger and William D. Fezler, in their book *Hypnosis and Behavior Modification: Imagery Conditioning* understand the use of suggestions during a normal hypnosis session for behavior modification. They said, "susceptibility to suggestion is apparently increased during hypnosis. This is one of the prime reasons for using it." In recall therapy, the information should come instead from the individual's recollection capabilities.

As we begin to understand the possibilities of layering, it becomes difficult to believe that the court system would allow any case to use a recalled image. It does not take much to taint any image. That is why, most often, regression or recall sessions involving serious implications are being done almost immediately to reduce the chance of images layered by a witness, family and friends. Some therapists even ask if the event has been discussed with other people before proceeding. They should!

"Memory is a complicated thing, a relative to truth, but not its twin."

-Barbara Kingsolver
Animal Dreams
(Harper Collins)

> "Originality does not consist in saying new things,
> but in treating old things in a new way."
>
> Goethe

CHAPTER THREE

IMPORTANCE OF SCRIPTING

Preparation for anything is important. As a therapist prepares his script and even conducts his sessions, no one looks over his shoulder except his own "Judge of Ethics."

Since wording is so important in hypnosis, putting those words together into a script carries the same value. Failure to overlook key words, phrases, times, emphases, and spacing can have a large impact on the success of the session.

Once the therapist has established the objective of the session in a prior meeting, he can begin to develop his script. If the client lists several objectives important to the session, the therapist should list them by priority. The questions on the therapist's script can begin to take shape based on that list. It is not important if the therapist has not covered all of the objectives in the allotted time. Other items on the list with less significance will provide a setting at a follow-up session. Of greatest importance to the client is the success of the session, and the first item on the list.

Therapists should always be cautious of regimented questions. "Regimented questions" are those that are so rehearsed that they completely ignore the response from a previous question. This happens when a therapist follows his script so intently that he does not listen to the response of the previous question. Writing a good script and rehearsing it well is a must if he is going to get through the session. However, the therapist's original script is not engraved in stone. It only provides a meaningful guide, a starting point. Once the session has begun, the therapist must be fluent enough to alter the next question based on his client's response. A good therapist must have the ability to listen intently to his client's every word while rewriting the Declaration of Independence during a session. Another challenge also exists. The therapist may have to skip the next question completely. That means he must remain flexible! Is this beginning to sound too complicated? Maybe it does to those who do not enjoy the challenge of discovery, or have the investigative nature about them, or who just want to know the results. The process should be exciting to the therapist also. When therapists fail to make it work and the love for this profession disappears, so will their clients.

WORDING

Words are important in effective communication in a normal state of consciousness, and twice as important in an altered state of consciousness. Simple words can make or break a hypnosis session. They can alter the course of the objective. They can intimidate the client to a point of no response, or they can be calming and effective.

"...and said unto the sea, Peace, be still. And the wind ceased, and there was a great calm."
Mark 4:39

Therapist's should have no doubt that they are in charge of the session and what they say; however they are not in charge of the individual's mind. The mind responds, based of years of information, to words spoken. Even a name is important. Let me give you an example. Although I have the individual's name in front of me, I always ask what name they prefer. It may be a nickname, or a comfortable name their family has called them for years. It may be the use of this name that makes them feel closer to the therapist. That closeness results in trust, and trust is important for a successful session.

For example, one client who visited me years ago had a first name of Lawrence. Most know that the nickname for Lawrence is Larry. However, family and friends always called him "Pud." That word change on the script made a tremendous difference. It also reinforced the trust, and made "Pud" comfortable. Without trust, the sessions would have been mediocre. With it, the session were limitless.

When therapists become extremely effluent with their script, they can improvise, make notes, or change the next question to coincide with the theme they are developing. It is important this task be accomplished while still listening carefully to each word being spoken by the client.

As we listen, we begin to interpret what we think was meant instead of clarifying by asking other questions. Not knowing what the client will say next, and to avoid leading, the therapist must remain flexible enough to alter the script at any given moment.

A typed script, rather than a hand written one, is easier to work with.   Add about two inches of space between questions.   This space gives enough area for notes or to rephrase the next question based on the response.   Notes or alterations may not be complete sentences, but they should provide enough information to formulate the next sentence quickly.

REHEARSAL

Most experts in the field emphasize the importance of voice and the natural flow of speech.   Stumbling over enunciation or pronunciation can cause the client's mind to drift, bringing the moment of the session back into the present.   We have all heard the phrase, "Practice what you preach."   Although this was not intended to mean practicing at rehearsals, it could not be more appropriate.

Know what to say and when.   Flexibility is important. Alertness plus flexibility allows therapists to make alterations. Therapists cannot be flexible if they do not have the basic script well rehearsed.   That does not mean the script must be memorized perfectly enough to present it at the next Kiwanis or Lion's club meeting.   Simply read it over several times.   Say it aloud and emphasize key words so the sentences flow naturally.   In essence, therapists are on stage.   Nobody wants the guiding to sound like a poorly practiced play.   Clients concentrate on the therapists words, or the way they pronounce words.   Many therapists have asked me to review recordings of sessions that did not seem to go well.   In most, the scripting was perfect.   However, some sounded like Bible-thumping preachers. Others sounded like the main speaker at the local high school graduation exercise. Their delivery was boring! Some therapists may get away with it occasionally, but the client can always detect boring. Winston Churchill's famous World War II quotation was "Never, never, never, never, give up!" Mine is "Practice, practice, practice, practice until you are comfortable."

"Whatever you would make habitual, practice it."

Epictetus

THE ART OF DESIGNING QUESTIONS

Designing proper questions is an art. Art enters design when therapists can satisfy both the "outsiders" and the client's objective. The outsiders are those individuals who are considering the client's recall as regressive testimony. Their satisfaction is important to a therapist's practice. It may be important, but is it important enough to lose sight of the client's objective for regression? Is it possible to satisfy the client's objective of unveiling the past and satisfying, too, the outsiders who are also interested? That is the art of designing questions.

Normally, we would consider only the objective of the client. However, in today's heightened awareness of childhood memories, the judicial system, lawsuits, criminal cases, abuse, past lives, age regression or even missing items, the careful phrasing of each sentence is important. There is no way of knowing when our questions will undergo scrutiny by other leading professionals or members of the court. Doing it right the first time is important, and a therapist should make it a habit to always do it correctly.

LEADING IS MISLEADING

We must fully understand "leading questions" and their impact. Each word a therapist interjects during the session can be leading, guiding or walking a client down an unfamiliar path. As he is being "mislead," his imagination and human responses create false memories. Ownership of those false memories belongs to the therapist, not the client.

Today, the public is willing to believe abuse accusations, no matter how meager the evidence. Our society has reached a point where some individuals consider it "in" to remember stories of childhood abuse, and some individuals have a need to be part of that scene. False memories may send innocent people to jail. Families suffer breakup, anger and legal battles, needlessly. Occasionally, the real perpetrator is the therapist. The American public is accepting as truth any allegations of abuse by therapists. It takes little evidence for a charge of abuse to surface. Even laws support this trend. The federal government has entered the picture. It developed the Child Abuse Prevention and Treatment Act. This Act requires health professionals, law enforcement officials, and educators to report suspected cases of abuse or face criminal penalties. It also promises the accusers immunity from prosecution if the reports prove false.

If a therapist triggers false memories in a client, he must be responsible for the consequences. Nothing exists to prevent the client from discussing the results with someone who falls under the umbrella of the Child Abuse Prevention and Treatment Act. Once that occurs, the therapist may become involved in a nasty court battle, whether he wants to be or not. The doors for a lawsuit are open if proof surfaces that the therapist has triggered false memories. The purpose of this book is to provide the therapist enough basic tools to prevent this story line from unfolding.

In trying to understand how false memories occur, we must realize that clients are interpreting every leading word, or series of words. We must also understand how emphasis and voice inflection can also be leading.

If a client uses a phrase to describe his own perception of a happening, when and if a pause permits, a therapist may question, "Who or what is behind that action?" His question is non threatening, non leading, is in alignment with the client's recounting. It also allows the client to continue on his train of thought and may offer additional information, useful to the regression.

Questioning errors creep into hypnotherapy sessions. Many therapists rely on their own "hunches" to get them through a recall session. These hunches are usually unsupported by valid reasons. We all come from various backgrounds, ethnic cultures, religions, environment, social and educational experiences. Because of these personal experiences we tend to jump to conclusions when judging people. We assume that their clothes, physical condition, speech, hair, color, eyes, shoes, hands, education or behavior pattern offers us an accurate portrait. It is this stereotyping that interferes with our questioning and may cause us to "lead" an individual down a path that may be unfamiliar territory. All therapists should be aware of tendencies to prejudge.

Sometimes, a client makes such a good or bad impression on us that we allow this to overshadow the moment. The therapist must not allow a personal relationship to develop between himself and a client, no matter how appealing, or beautiful, or interesting, or rich and famous the client is. Therapists should remain objective and treat everyone the same. The rich and the beautiful deserve no better than the ugly and smelly. All therapists need to strive for objectivity in their judgment of clients. Concentrate on concrete observations. Monitor behavior during the pre-induction interview. Observe body language and verbal statements, looking for consistency between the two. Look for signs of anxiety, poor self-esteem, positive attitude, happiness or uncertainties. Concentrate more on what they say and do than on their clothes, jewelry and occupation.

Therapists should always create a pleasant atmosphere. They should greet all clients warmly and do everything to put them at ease.

During the pre induction interview, the therapist should explain exactly what is going to take place so the client will not experience any surprises. Ask what his friends call him, and if you may do the same. Try to create a friendly, relaxed atmosphere.

The following list provides a beginning compilation of guidelines that may be helpful in regressive hypnosis sessions.

● Try not to interrupt the client during a session.

● Never question the response. Allow him the freedom to describe what he is seeing, feeling, experiencing or touching.

● Never express surprise or disapproval or dismay.

● Never cross examine the client -- he may freeze up.

● Never try to rush a client. Scheduling recall sessions as the last appointment for the day is wise. It will reduce the chances of normal office interruptions.

● Never judge.

● Never "break in" at a pause in the response. If the client has not responded after a fifteen or 20-second break, the therapist may come to his assistance with the next "non leading" question. In a normal conversation between two people we anticipate a response. During a recall session, knowing when to intervene usually separates the professional therapist from the amateur.

● Never ask a question without a clear purpose in mind.

● Avoid awkward pauses on your part. Be prepared. Therapists should place their script in front of them. Listen to the response. Time any pauses. State your next question in words that parallel the moment.

● Remember, interpretation of response is not the function of a therapist until all the data has been collected. Then the results may be analyzed.

Are there traits that therapists should possess or try to develop? Definitely! They should possess the ability to improvise. A professional therapist must be patient, warm, and excel in thoroughness. He should be non analytical, non judgmental, organized, rational, unassuming, and familiar with the objective. Above all, he should be a good listener, meticulous, tolerant, and flexible. Every therapist should be intelligent, sensitive, practical, self disciplined, and he should, above all, love people.

Always take control. Obtain the information wanted within a reasonable time. A professional can accomplish this without interfering with the client's spontaneity of response. He must use a permissive approach allowing free recall of memories, or he may lose the real purpose. The balance of control over the session is in his hands.

It is difficult, but therapists must learn to determine the end of the client's response. With time and practice it becomes easier.

Leading questions cause a client unintentionally to structure his memory toward what he thinks will please the therapist. They also let the client know what the therapist considers to be a favorable response. Leading questions keep accurate information from surfacing.

All questions should be "open-ended" and should not suggest the most desirable response. Open-ended questions do not ask for a definite reply. They cannot be answered with a simple "yes," or "no." They may take on the form of, "Tell me more about that." This type of questioning allows a person to recall in greater detail without trying to satisfy a particular therapist's likes or dislikes.

A "depth question" requires a little more analysis of the recalled scene. "Could you tell me where you are? Could you describe what is taking place?"

The approach is different if they are trying to describe the size of an object. After they say something is large and a therapist has waited a reasonable amount of time, asking is permissible if questioning is noncommittal as, "It is as large as what?"

The therapist should not worry whether or not others understand leading questions, especially those in the legal profession. The judicial system of this country understands leading questions. The subject of leading questions is a constant challenge to attorneys. Most of the challenges are based on a single word, or emphasis on a word. The difference in hypnosis recall is simple. All questions should undergo a once-over by the therapist before they ever reach a court of law. Each therapist has an obligation as a professional to scrutinize each question they ask during a session. They owe that protection to their client as well.

THE POWER OF WORDS

A mind is like wet cement; whatever the therapist says may make a lasting impression. During the opening discussion or in the actual hypnosis session the impression may deepen with the manner in which each word is spoken.

When we hear a word, it triggers an inner response. We search our memory bank for a definition. The process occurs in nanoseconds. During the search process we even compare the word with the process wherein we learned it. We also check on what it means to us intellectually and emotionally. Let me give an example.

If I speak the word "sex" each of us automatically begins a process of recall. To some, the word may carry a negative connotation. Others may attach a meaning that carries exciting and wonderful implications. To a particular single female client, it may mean abstinence. Yet, to a particular male client, it may trigger an intense inner discomfort recalling impotence. Another may visualize it as a time his mother or father beat him when he was discovered exploring his own body as a child. Yet, to some, the word may mean beautiful nude forms, the softness of flesh, sighs of contentment, exuberance and pleasure. It may mean babies, children and stressful responsibilities. It may mean control over others, or a way to earn an income. Even a small word like "sex" and its personal connotations can take on infinitesimal interpretations.

Words have power. They can be magical or they can be manipulative. Written or spoken, words have the power to build up or tear down. They have the power to set people free or to imprison them. Proper word choice is a long learning process. It takes reading, and practice. This exploration into the use of words also includes the process of how we express ourselves. Learning to express ourselves properly takes time. Therapists can do it. The first step in any process is to be aware of the power of words.

Wherefore comfort one another with these words.
1 Thessalonians 4:18

The lyrics of many songs remind us to "emphasize the positive, delete the negative..." This is great advice for lovers and parents, for teachers, bosses, and especially for therapists. Negativity can destroy a perfect session. Negative words carry such an impact by reinforcing a client's bad habits or behaviors.

The ability to detect words of a negative nature in a conversation can quickly aid in a therapist's analysis of an individual's character. Sensitivity to negative language becomes a trait that is extremely useful, in relationships, business, and family.

The client's constant use of negative words during a session can be a process of denial. Nothing constructive can surface in a barrage of negative words. The use of negative words or phrasing by therapists interferes with the client's need for positive reinforcement. He came seeking assistance in making positive changes in behavior and habits.

Most of us can get all the negativity we want at home, work or socializing. The mere indication that someone is going to a therapist and will be using hypnosis to recall a childhood event will surface negativity.   It often will bring out the worst from coworkers, friends and family members:

"I went once and it **didn't** work for me."

"Oh, you can do it on your own, you **don't** need therapy or hypnosis."

"I'll bet they **can't** hypnotize you."

"If you discover something, you **won't** do anything about it."

"You **won't** be able to recall all of your childhood."

"I'll bet you **haven't** told your family about all of this."

"I **never** did believe in that stuff."

"Well, **don't** expect any support from me."

The universe is bombarding us all the time with negativity. **Don't** get too fat! **Don't** hit your sister! **No** dogs allowed. **Don't** rain on my parade! **Don't** touch, **don't** laugh, **don't** cry, **don't** walk and **do not** pass go. It is all around us, reinforcing negative attitudes. The bombardment surfaces in a variety of forms. Stopping your car at a stop sign without confronting some sort of negativity is almost impossible. Maybe it is the impatience of the person in the car behind you. Maybe it is the car in front of you displaying a bumper sticker that reads, "Mother-in-law in truck!" The bumper sticker may be funny to some, but it is still part of the bombardment. The little bumper sticker is just one of a thousand signs, displays, TV shows, movies, advertisement, news, interviews, and even clothing that becomes part of the barrage of negativity. Do these torpedo our minds in the light of good humor as their creators meant, or do we store them in our memory bank, reinforcing our own negativity?

Clients need strong affirmations and positive reinforcement. They need to hear someone constantly affirming their objectives and how they can accomplish them. Clients need to hear that they carry beliefs that interfere with their ability to move forward. They do not need to hear it through a process of adding more "Thou shalt not's."

"...but say in a word, and my servant shall be healed."

Luke 7:7

To remove negativity completely, we must all learn to rephrase all statements so that the negative words disappear from our speech patterns. What are a few of the words to watch for?

No	mustn't	don't	can't
never	won't	shouldn't	wouldn't

CHOOSING OUR WORDS WISELY

All therapists using hypnosis should know their boundaries on word usage. They should know where traveling is safe. Therapists should increase their awareness of word usage. That does not necessarily mean adding more words to our vocabulary. It simply means the careful usage of words we all use on a daily basis. Each therapist should be sensitive enough to tune into the client's response. Each should monitor his own behavior in the use of negative words at home and in social settings. The average child, from birth until the time he or she enters first grade has heard the word **"No"** more than forty thousand times. How many "no's" and "wont's" and "cant's" can our minds take? Whatever the limit is, a therapist can avoid compounding the situation.

The use of negative words during a session may add to the triggering of false memories. Any negative response to what the client is experiencing in a recall mode can completely change the images. Researchers have discovered that the use of other biased or "colored" words can influence an individual's interpretation of an event, whether it is in either short term or long term memory storage. This type of information is important in a court of law.

Nationally, several universities made a commitment to

study the impact of words and their usage. The results were astounding. Volunteers agreed to watch a motion picture film involving an automobile accident. After watching the film, each received these instructions: They had just witnessed an accident and their recollection of the event was extremely important. Each answered the same basic question. Unbeknownst to the volunteers, researchers conducting the study were changing only the verb of the sentence. The original question was, "About how *fast* were the cars going when they *hit* each other?" The interviewers substituted the word *hit* with such words as: smashed, collided, bumped or contacted. Individual recollection was altered according to the specific word used, as well as their estimation of the speed of the car. Some varied as much as ten miles an hour.

The experiment continued with another question, "Did you see *a* broken headlight?" Others received a revised question; "Did you see *the* broken headlight?" The question that uses *the* infers a broken headlight exists. The question that uses the word *a* really makes no definite statement one way or another. It does not even imply that the headlight is broken. If a tiny word like *the* can lead people to recall something they never saw, what about the bigger words we use during recall? What we remember, it seems, may not be exactly what happened and therapists should remain "hidden observers.".

Recently, an article published in *The Lancet*, a English medical journal, verified a story of an individual who caused his own death because of the words he saw. The patient discovered that he had a form of leukemia by looking at his doctor's notes over his shoulder. The doctor had never told him his was a very mild form, or explained his condition, including that he was likely to live for many years. The man missed his next doctor's visit and died weeks later, apparently from neglecting himself. Even an autopsy failed to explain the man's rapid decline.

"How sweet are thy words unto my taste! yea, sweeter than honey to my mouth! Through thy precepts I get understanding: therefore I hate every false way. Thy word is a lamp unto my feet, and a light unto my path."

Psalm 119:103-105

To understand how differences take form we must first try to grasp the storage process of the mind. Memory researchers know we store words as symbols. Each stored word means different things to different people. The following is a short list of words that take on an individual meaning. This simple exercise provides a better understanding of perception. Understanding the process can drastically reduce the surfacing of false memories triggered by therapists. Each word, and its meaning as stored by the client, may show great differences from meanings in the mind of the therapist. That is something that we must accept and understand. We should recall a picture for each symbol, and ask ourselves, as we repeat the following words: could our image be different from our client's image?

fence	warm	sex	teacher
furniture	cold	sexual	principal
hedge	pain	water	money
scale	pressure	bizarre	vase
doll	car	truck	drum
brick	lamp	shore	road

A word could be a starting point for accuracy. It could also be a starting point for catastrophic deterioration. The senses provide the raw information. Individual perception gives meaning to what we see, hear, taste, and smell.

"Things are to me as they appear to me, and to you as they appear to you, and no ground exists for saying that one opinion is any truer than the other."

Plato

We can release a flow of healing power by the words we speak. Words can change the atmosphere of both business and home. Negative or careless words have the power to destroy. Words of hope and praise have the power to build up.

During the pre induction interview therapists can plant seeds of doubt and despair in the hearts of their clients. They have the power of speaking hope to hearts that may be hurting or are in need of encouragement. Aeschylus said, "Words are the physicians of a mind diseased." All therapists should speak words of affirmation. They must remember that a thoughtful word is like a refreshing drink of water to a weary desert traveler.

IMPORTANT KEY WORDS

Key words can provide the therapist an avenue for information. They also allow the client the freedom to create, explore, recall, experience, expand, develop, or describe a person, place, thing or event. If the therapist is using key words incorrectly, they can also trigger false memories, confusion, layered images, discomfort, disorientation and chaos.

It was the film actor Mickey Rooney who said, "On

this planet, age is nothing more than experience, so some of us are just more experienced than others." Based on his analogy, the experienced therapists might remember comedian Flip Wilson whose famous phrase was, "What you see is what you get." In recall sessions, it is "what you say is what you get." If the therapist speaks the "precise" key word, he will get "precisely" what he asked for.

In the section *The Power of Words*, we learn that each word triggers a personal interpretation and meaning. Now, we will approach the avoidance of personal interpretation by using key words. The objective is to learn how to select key words that prevent clients from any inner interpretation based solely on wording. The experienced therapist will allow them to explore the regression and experience the moment without triggering false memories.

When a client is in any regressive state of consciousness, the therapist should always be specific in his questioning. However, some specific words may be leading, or misleading. Our goal then is to select certain words that will suffice as a replacement to avoid that catastrophe.

Examples appear to explain any situation better than theory. In reference books on the subject of hypnosis, many authors allude to specific wording during a recall session. They outline their style of questioning in great detail. Developing a style is wonderful, however, focusing on wording is even more important. Those associated with hypnosis all began using standard scripts in daily sessions. The scripts provided the therapists a common ground as they began using hypnosis as a valuable tool. Sometimes they used the provided scripts because of the author's success, or they began using them simply because they were there, and they did not have to develop scripts of their own. There are pitfalls within the borders of those standard scripts. Now is the time for therapists to alter, design, and develop sound personal scripts, flexible enough to withstand a viable session, and the possibility of news media and judicial scrutiny.

The following is an example of the type of scenario to avoid during a regression, and the reasons why.

"Look around the room."

"Look at the pictures on the wall, the items on the shelves and tables in the room."

"Does any of it look familiar?"

Those questions appear harmless, but are they? We are making an assumption that the client has already stated that he is in a room. That may sound silly, but if the therapist is not paying attention to responses, the next question may be out of order.

The next sentence is where the "leading" begins. When the therapist instructs him to, "Look at the pictures on the wall, the items on the shelves and tables in the room," the therapist has inadvertently taken the lead. This kind of wording is based on the broad assumption that everyone has pictures on the walls and items on tables in every room. However, by inserting those innocent words, the process of instruction has begun. Any kind of instruction places the therapist in the lead role. The client's response may be a response on the instructions, not his own visual recognition.

The passive approach, using different wording, would remove any fear of leading. "Would you mind describing to me what you see in the room and on the walls?" Asking if he minds describing what he sees avoids the lead. We know walls exist, or he would not have described it as a room. It also allows him freedom to scan and interrupt his visualization. It offers an opportunity to express to the best of his recollection. He has another option. Maybe he does not want to share the information with the therapist. Of course, we want him to share the information and chances are, he will. Offering the client an option to use his own trust and judgment is a powerful tool for accuracy. He already has a certain amount of trust in this therapy or he would not be submitting to hypnosis. He is aware of the therapist's presence and feels comfortable and trusting. He is usually willing to describe to the therapist what he sees. It is up to the therapist to then follow his response with another non leading question.

"Are you experiencing any emotions and feelings being in the room?"

If the response is positive, the therapist may follow with, "Would you share your feelings and emotions with me?" Some have referred to this type of questioning as passive. It is. Many consider this passive approach as "non leading," and that is important when dealing with memories. The client has an understanding that he can share what he sees and feels. The more he shares the more he trusts. The more he trusts, the more sensitive the therapist must become of transference and its complications. (See Section on *Transference*.) The more he trusts and feels comfortable with the therapist exploring his memory bank, the more he shares and the better the recall. A good recall session means the therapist accomplished the task. Any practitioner of hypnosis will feel a sense of pride knowing that everything was done without leading.

CHAPTER FOUR

THE INDUCTION

Induction techniques vary as do the personalities of therapists. However, the environment during a recall induction is different from other sessions. Recall sessions have a high tendency of inquiry. Behavioral therapy sessions are addressing behavior of a client. A difference exists between these two types of sessions and the same principles do not apply. As professionals, all therapists should understand the difference. Any therapist may use a standard induction technique to obtain a state of relaxation and responsiveness. Even then, therapists should take the time to initiate a self examination to make sure the induction is free of any leading. Therapists should screen everything they do. If it is free of any interference, they may continue the session as usual. If it is not, they should rewrite and make the changes now. However, once the individual has reached the state of suggestibility, the therapist's involvement must change.

After the initial induction during a recall session, the therapist must take on the role as an observer, not a participant. Let the client establish the scene, do not lead him into one. If therapists provide leading questions during recall sessions, chances are good that they will become active participants. Their degree of participation may not be exactly what they had in mind. The therapist may unwittingly become a defendant in a court of law, or the subject of an expose on the front page of the *National Enquirer*. This type of public exposure can be damaging to both client and therapist. A little extra care may save a professional career from embarrassment.

PASSIVE INDUCTION

I believe that is important to digress at this time and discuss "Passive Induction." Passive induction allows a client to be more submissive with the information he provides. If obtained using passive induction, the information provided during a recall session offers a client the discretion or decision to view, recall, define or experience the moment. We cannot ignore the probability that the information gathered during a passive induction may be acceptable in a court of law. In a passive induction, information offered is that of the client and not the opinion of the therapist.

I realize that many therapists do not use passive inductions during other types of sessions. However, I strongly suggest consideration in using this approach during a recall. During smoking cessation sessions, for example, therapists may use techniques that are stronger-acting to support their purpose. In recall sessions, therapists provide a path in seeking specifics. If the therapist breaks the chain, he will simply have two pieces of chain, not an accuracy of recollection. In this circumstance, he should pretend he is Mahatma Gandhi, and be passive. Like Gandhi, it will get him further in his objectives.

LOOKING FOR BLAME

Therapists should never lose sight of *their client's purpose*. They should mutually discuss that purpose thoroughly before beginning any session dealing with memories. If the client cannot readily define his purpose, he may be looking for a scape goat. He may already be into blame, and in fact, may be ready to obtain information through a recall session to sue, file charges or expose someone.

Today, therapists will confront individuals who, instead of taking responsibility for their own lives, feel compelled to blame their troubles on someone else. If they can blame another person, they will never need to change themselves. To some, identifying and solving the real problem is not important. They are only anxious to shift the burden of responsibility to someone else.

During all opening discussions, therapists should ask themselves, "Does my client have destructive patterns or characteristics?" "Are they stuck on blame and externalizing?" (Externalizing is the process of believing that something "out there" is always the reason for their difficulties. Externalizing is what some people do to relieve their pain. It is their means of escape.) "I will feel better if I blame someone, take drugs, or drink."

If some of these patterns surface, therapists should ask themselves,

"Does my client need to feel loved by someone?"

"Does she have a compelling need to change others?"

"Does she have a need to always be right?"

"Does she need to be constantly in control?"

"After these sessions, can she move forward in her life?"

"Is she rational?"

If a therapist feels unqualified, or untrained, to interpret those feelings and emotions, then he should recommend the client to someone who is trained to do so. Sometimes, individuals may have justification for blame. However, therapists must be careful not to be a factor in adding false blame.

Many individuals sincerely want to discover an event from their past that they feel controls their present life. The therapist must then decide whether the trip is worth their reputation. Each therapist must decide if a possibility exists that the search is going to uncover old garbage that may put him on the witness stand. Will the old garbage result in his trying to defend himself, his business and his profession? He must decide if these serious and deep-seated conflicts are something that he feels he can, or even wants to handle. If his feelings are borderline, then the client should referred to an expert on that subject.

Many individuals have more difficulty in accepting their life than in making changes. They have difficulty realizing that sometimes it is more beneficial to simply accept the past, recognize it as such, then move forward. I have always displayed an old metaphysical saying on my office wall, hoping that some may read it and accept it: These are the ten most powerful two-letter words in the English language. "If it is to be, it is up to me."

Case in point. A young lady, probably in her middle thirties, scheduled an appointment. During our opening discussion, (I do not like to use the term "pre-talk." Some therapists use that term and some schools teach those words as an intricate part of a session. However, to me it means "before talking" which I interrupt to mean a study of the client's body language.) spoke of a tragedy that occurred when she was a child. Her family refused to discuss it. She felt she played a major role in the event and wanted to experience an age regression to discover exactly what took place. I asked for more details.

She told me that at the age of four, she and her little sister (three years of age) went exploring an empty house near their home. She recalled coming out of the building with blood splattered all over her white dress. No other children or adults were around. Her little sister died. She wanted a recall session to see if she caused her death.

I thought about several factors. If I took her back and she recalled the event in detail, what impact would it have on her life? Could her family, who had been covering up this horrendous event, possibly sue me for exposing the tragedy? Is there a point when not knowing all of the particulars is better than knowing? Could she handle the consequences if she was responsible for the death?

I ask her how important it was for her to know for sure? She hesitated, then said, "I *think* I want to know."

Based on her use of the word "think," I opened the discussion further. When someone uses the word *think*, they may be unsure. Here, the pain of knowing could be the uncertainty. The pain of taking the responsibility could be the reason for her indecision.

I said, "Whatever happened may or may not be important. That is for you to decide. Before you decide, I would like you to consider something. If you do go back and recall the event in detail, you must remember that whatever took place was between a three year-old and four year-old. The mind of a four-year-old has not fully developed her bank of knowledge. A four-year-old has not learned all of the principles of life. She does not understand danger. She does not fully understand the consequences of her actions. Children watch a cartoon and see their favorite mouse character smack the bad cat on the head with a hammer. The bad cat shakes his head, a goose egg appears and then the chase is on again. A four-year-old experiments with life, which is how we learn. A strong possibility exists that some sort of accident did occur. Even if you did something that resulted in your little sister's death, it was still an accident. A child's memory bank is very small. A four-year-old has not had that much experience."

I went on to say, "What a four-year-old, did or did not do, is difficult for a thirty-five-year-old person to take the responsibility for. In fact, it is almost impossible to comprehend. A four-year-old may not want to hurt her little sister, but maybe a game went too far. Just like the television cartoons, would a simple push or a "bonk" on the head hurt anyone? Do you really want to know what that little girl did? Do you want to carry around guilt from the action of a four-year-old mind?"

She thought for a few minutes before I continued.

"Please do yourself, me and your family a favor. Take the next couple of weeks to think about this. If at the end of the two weeks you still want to pursue it, I will schedule a session." She thanked me and left.

Two weeks later I received a call from the young lady. She told me she never felt better in her life. She said she understood what I had said in our conversation. She knew that at the age of thirty-five she could not possibly take a life, however, as a little four-year-old she could possibly have made a mistake. She had talked over her decision with the family and was comfortable for the first time in her life. She could not thank me enough for her progress. I explained that her progress was her own doing. We decided to abandon the recall session, to avoid bringing up old pain, guilt and family discomfort. The catalyst my concern was simply her use of the word "think."

Experiencing growth is difficult, unless we let go of old garbage from the past. When individuals withhold emotions they deplete their energy, leaving them physically, spiritually and emotionally bankrupt! Therapists should talk to their clients about learning to express emotions honestly, openly, and appropriately. They should focus on the person rather than the process. Listen to what they are saying. Therapists have the power to prevent molehills from growing into mountains.

NONVERBAL COMMUNICATION CAN TRIGGER FALSE MEMORIES

Nonverbal communication can trigger false memories. Memories receive a certain amount of influence, if they are not completely changed, when exposed to nonverbal communication with others. Children's responses to a parent can be, and are usually, based around the body language of that parent. When a parent is questioning a child about a wrong doing, the child will, unknowingly, alter his story based on the parent's body language. The folded arms and stern look of a towering mother can instill a quick fabrication from a child as he recalls the events that led to a broken window. The child's recall of the event is altered slightly as he begins layering new scenes on top of the original.

Nonverbal communication in therapy can, and often does, have the same effect. One of the most publicized cases of childhood memories of sexual abuse, involving small children and a father, occurred in Utah. It became a "witch hunt" of great proportions. Publicly, the attention often revolves around the father, the children, or the therapist working with the violated children. The media tried and sentenced the Utah father before the case ever went to trial. The state of Utah responded swiftly.

Because of heavy case loads, contracting therapy and counselors is common for States. Utah is no different. Most of the Utah population was not aware of these "contracted services" until this case. It opened the eyes of many therapists. It also took a hard look at the manner in which therapists ask questions.

The therapist involved in this particular case had won the contract awarded by the state shortly before the case broke into the news. State officials decided to assign her this case based on her success with this type of recall. The father's guilt or innocence was not the point. The method of recall was most important.

This case brought national attention to a small town outside Salt Lake City, Utah. The father, a respected member of the community and active church member, was charged with sexual abuse of his two little daughters. The town was devastated. The townspeople took up sides.

The news media played havoc with everyone concerned. They interviewed anyone who had contact with any member of the family.   They aired interviews with neighbors, friends, school teachers and church leaders. Their coverage even included the school crossing guard. The news media became the judge, jury and court. Their broadcasts filled all of the local affiliates. National television networks jumped on the wagon. Later, the Public Broadcast System (PBS) used the video coverage. The PBS producers later aired the case and information when they included it as part of a series on sexual abuse discoveries. Within a short period, accusations surfaced against other fathers. The witch hunt was on. Later, authorities dropped the charges against the other fathers.

Most ignored what was taking place in private. What was happening to the children involved in the case? Was the contracted therapist doing a good job? State officials became concerned at the constant coverage on national television. They decided to investigate and monitor the contracted therapist. One psychiatrist received the assignment for this task. After monitoring the procedures from the safety of a two-way mirror, the state psychiatrist reported, in disbelief, the unethical tactics of the therapist. The officials refused to listen or to do anything about it.   The well known and respected state psychiatrist turned in his resignation. What was the contracted therapist doing that caused a man of this stature to walk away from a well paying job?

The contracted therapist was to obtain statements for the prosecution from the children involved. What the states psychiatrist witnessed and reported was the method of questioning being used by the therapist. He reported that the female therapist would position herself and the child on a large quilt in the center of the floor. She used a baby doll for the child to point where the her father had touched her. The use of a baby doll is an acceptable practice. Often, it is the recommended procedure. The doll provides a process so therapists do not lead the child. Placing words into the child's thought pattern by recommending a part of the body is very easy. The use of a doll prevents this from happening. So far, the action by the therapist was routine. The action that followed shocked the psychiatrist. The therapist would question the child and wait for a verbal response, or she would, herself, point to a part of the baby doll. The unethical procedures entered the picture with the physical response (nonverbal communication) of the therapist.

If the therapist did not like the response, she would fold her arms and turn her back on the little child. If she approved what the child said or where she pointed, she would scoop up the child into her arms, and tell the child how well she had done. Even the unpolluted mind of a small child can figure out the procedure that best serves her. The child was learning "a conditioned response to a conditioned stimulus." Since this process is repetitive, the mind of a small child forms new images. Eventually, it would be almost meaningless in a court of law, to ask a child to recall the original image without the benefit of hypnosis. (See the Section on Layering)

The therapist, an attractive woman, became the center of the controversy surrounding this case. Male therapists joked about the case saying, "I'll tell her anything if she'll pick me up and hug me."

Acceptance was important to these children. That response was childlike in nature. Torn from their family, the children began to question their values. The news media was hunting them down like animals, and they could not see their mother or other relatives. How should a child alone and confused respond to affection and approval? Each of us would probably respond the same way.

Whether the therapist believed in her techniques is immaterial for this discussion. What is important is an understanding as to how nonverbal communication can influence recall. The children involved here may never know, and may never recall the original memories without the use of properly induced hypnosis. New images, have become a part of their recall process. Their false memories, permeated by the body language of a therapist, became part of the court's documents. They found the father guilty. True or untrue, no one will ever know for sure.

If the accusation by the state's investigator was true, a single therapist's actions affected many people. The domino effect took its toll and will linger for years. The state lost a brilliant and concerned psychiatrist by refusing to investigate his accusations and accepting his resignation. A father went to jail. A family, and the lives of their relatives and friends, will never be the same. Some good news did come out of this unpleasantness. The state of Utah now monitors contracts differently. Other states learned a valuable lesson. If you are going to look for the bad news, you do not have to look far. The entire episode brought more unanswered questions to light. Did the notoriety and publicity engulf the therapist so much that it may have drawn in her own ego? Was the court wrong to allow the children's testimony after it became aware of the therapist's behavioral techniques? Was the court system aware of the accusations? If they were aware, were the accusations true? Did the court system get so caught up in the momentum of the witch hunt that they wanted to set an example? Was the father guilty? We will never know for sure. What we do know is that nonverbal communication, however subtle, plays a vital role in behavior, response to others behavior, and subsequently affects memories.

From the moment the client meets the therapist, he is

analyzing the therapist's body language. He is analyzing nonverbal communication, not on a professional level but on a subconscious level. He is analyzing it on the same level as the small child who is confronting his mother about a broken window.

Acceptance is important to everyone. During the 'pre induction' visit, the individual is looking for the therapist's acceptance. How the therapist responds initially may set the mood for the entire session. That includes the therapist's body language. The therapist's nonverbal communication to the client is important. It may determine the mood, and whether they are comfortable enough to be completely open.

Unlike the therapist in the Utah case, most therapists do not know whether their cases will end in a court of law. Whatever the outcome, use common sense. All therapists should learn the basics of nonverbal communication. It is part of the client - therapist process.

LEADING

If therapists are going to dance with the past utilizing hypnosis, they should not take the lead! That may sound like a silly statement, but I mean it in all seriousness. Sometimes therapists may think a question is great without really examining its content, word power and legalities. This type of self scrutiny is important to both the client and the therapist. We all need to remind ourselves that the mind becomes creative with very little information. With the planting of a seed, the mind automatically takes over and enhances the therapist's leading question, resulting in false memories. Certain questions may trigger a belief that results in high stress, psychological problems, undue pain and suffering. Investigators have traced the destruction of families, criminal charges, law suits and even the loss of businesses to fabricated memories resulting from leading questions. False memories have led to divorce, allowed the release of child molesters and murderers, imprisonment of innocent people and the loss of homes. The list of devastation is endless.

Maybe the title of this book should have been, "Before you lead your client, know what kind of suit you want to wear in court."

This is serious business. No therapist has a right to lead a client! If therapists develop an internal excitement based on some of their clients' responses, they should be apprehensive. Therapists who are starting to feel intrigued by their client's response may be beginning to lead subconsciously. That is when our own fantasies enter the session. It happens. Sometimes it is a struggle not to be inquisitive. Some therapists act as if it is a waste of time if they do not break the story of the century by creating false memories within their client. Others are constantly looking for sensationalism. In that search, they feel they will enhance their ego if they can unlock blocked memories from the past. Therapists must constantly remind themselves that it is the clients' past and not their own.

All therapists should review their list of questions. If they have doubts, that is a good sign they are sensitive to the situation. I have included some questions therapists may ask themselves as they review their list of questions. This list will become automatic with experience. They should take their time with the questions until they are comfortably secure with them. The best therapists have made mistakes. Across the nation, some leading therapists have inadvertently ignored their list of questions only to have solid cases thrown out of court or have found themselves facing serious charges. All therapists should take time to review the following list.

"Is the question leading?" Is the client placed in a situation, relationship, or environment that has the possibility of being interpreted as leading?

"Does it instill inappropriate thoughts?" Does the question lead him into a circumstance that may be inappropriate for his sex, age, circumstance or values?

"Have I instilled false ideas in my client by my wording or phraseology?" Analyze each word for its meaning. As the therapist, did you possibly use a word that is misappropriate in this circumstance? What kind of power is behind each word?

"Would a judge, in a court of law, accept the question?" Would those from the legal profession believe that you are not leading the client? Has your phrasing allowed for freedom to recall events, places, things or people on their own? Have you omitted words that may influence description of events, places, things or people?

"Have I injected my own thoughts?" Did I mistakenly think that the client meant something he did not mean? As he used particular words that meant subjective things to him, did I automatically assume it to mean something different?

"Did I interpret his responses wrong during our opening discussion?" Did the clients use of a certain word trigger some of my own biases? Are we on the same wavelength? Should I clarify before we begin any session?

When a therapist provides his or her own thoughts as to the outcome, it becomes a premise. This assumption has resulted in many ill-fated sessions. It is ill-fated especially when the client's recollection has not revealed a comparable situation. If a therapist presumes anything, he has opened the door to devastation and ridicule for both his client and himself. Every childhood problem, for example, does not stem from sexual abuse. The same regression, aided by two different therapists, can have different results due only to the design of questions.

The real tragedies of this scenario are the legalities involved. Without leading them, therapists should have their clients produce solid, accurate, information. This is the goal of all professional therapists, or should be.

LEADING QUESTIONS AND MISPLACED ITEMS

Someone once said to me that "Leading questions and misplaced items," should be the title of a country - western song. It could be, except these two subjects, leading questions and misplaced items, go together like the pope and gambling.

Some clients are looking for missing items. Without the proper use of hypnosis the chances of finding them may be very slim. Properly placed questions during recall can frequently surface the location of the missing item..

The search for misplaced items can be a tedious process. The demand for patience on the therapist is high. Any assistance offered by the therapist is a hindrance. The client adapts to the interference and accepts the fact that the therapists knows where the item is. They will follow the guidance of the therapist on a path to nowhere.

The therapist should learn to keep out of the way. The client knows what the item is and eventually will recall where she placed it. The mind recorded all of the information, and it can easily recall that event. Using one or more of the senses, the mind can recall, duplicate, and place the client back into the original setting. Unless someone exterior to the minds' workings interjects an alternative thought that interferes, the client's ability to recall should work wonderfully.

The search for misplaced items is fascinating. It is like being part of a mystery. Therapists are monitoring the search of a treasured family heirloom, a paycheck, vacation money or the keys to the summer cabin. Being part of the mystery does not include utterance of any words that would create new images in the mind of the searcher.

The therapist should have the client recall and describe the item in precise detail. While in a state of hypnosis, she should describe the size, shape, color and weight of the item for which she is searching. If it was a gift, the therapist should ask if she would mind sharing who gave it to her, and when. Each of these types of questions interacts with the memory storage process and brings the image of the item forward so she can deal with it. The detailed description is an important function in the chain of memory recall.

The therapist should ask her to recall approximately the last time she saw or handled the item. Sometimes, the very act of recalling the last time she had it adds drastically to the process of recall. Possession triggers the physical sense, an aspect of recall that summons the feel, touch, weight and shape of the item. Possession of the item may also place her into a particular time frame. That may be the clue to narrow down the time into the crucial segment. To enhance the process further, the therapist should ask if she recalls the approximate hour she was in possession of or saw the item. Avoid asking her the "time-of-day." The word "day" signifies daylight to most people, and unless the therapist is conducting his session at the north pole, in actuality, the time of the incident may have been during the hours of darkness. Listen carefully to the wording.

Descriptions of a room, item, house, furniture, garden, etc. are important. Listen to each word. Occasionally, I even draw the layout of the room as the details are recalled. The therapist is working for a detective mind.

I once figured out the time of day by the client's description of the room. She followed the description by adding that the morning sun entered the windows on the left side. Knowing where she was standing, the direction she was facing and the direction of the house, figuring it out that it was during the morning hours was easy. The early morning sun would enter those particular windows. As she spoke she began recalling the fine details of the room and the position of the morning sun. She even mentioned how the early morning sun reflected off the fish aquarium on the opposite side of the room.

I am offering a word of caution. The therapist has already begun to trigger false memories if he asks, "Was it morning?" A simple injection of the word "morning" has placed the client in a specific time of day and that may not have been the time the event took place. The therapist has interrupted the flow of thoughts with the use of one simple word.

The word "morning" carries a powerful meaning to each of us. It began to shape when we were in diapers. Our learning process is cumulative. "Morning" carried specific meanings to us as children, and expanded as we grew older. Today, when we hear that word our minds automatically collect all of those stored images and links them with accompanying feelings and emotions. (See Section on Layering)

If, when asking a client to describe the item, the therapist interjects his own thoughts, he might as well end the session. For example, if we are looking for a set of keys to the summer cabin, each of us speculates on what a set of keys looks like. We, as therapists, are no different from other people. We immediately imagine the misplaced key ring with several keys on the ring. Inadvertently, we may even picture a lucky charm or something attached to it. We probably would not stop there. We would add color, weight and size. Helping by describing the item if the client is having difficulty or is slow in responding seems very natural. Sometimes, trying to be helpful, we can be so unhelpful.

In a normal conversation, we automatically finish or want to finish a sentence for people who hesitate. We also have learned that sometimes people expect us to finish their sentences. It is no different in a session. The tendency to help, and to complete sentences or thoughts, still surfaces, although it has no business in a hypnosis session. Each therapist has a responsibility to suppress on the natural tendency to intervene. Intervention can mean a scattered session. Once the images become diffused with new thoughts, it is almost impossible to return to the original purpose.

Be careful and listen to responses to questions. Ask neutral questions (See the Section on Neutral questions). Learn to be an outsider looking in, not an active participant in the search.

ARE YOU LISTENING?

Do therapists listen? Really listen? Listening is one of the most ignored aspects of regressive therapy. Current schools and classes that teach hypnosis seem to bypass this subject. Yet, if therapists plan to excel in this field, they must train themselves to be good listeners.. Without it, they will continue to maintain a mediocre status. Without it, fate will have them creating false memories.

People crave someone to listen to them, probably more than anything else in their life. Listening is 50 percent of good communication. Communication fails if listening is absent. If therapists do not have good communication in their relationships, in marriage, business, service, friendships, and with their children, they have managed to be mediocre in all aspects of their life.

Why do radio and television personalities excel as interviewers, broadcasters and talk-show hosts? Johnny Carson, Dick Cavet, Connie Chung, David Frost, and Sally Jessie Raphael all have a commonality. They all are masters at listening. They can alter their questions, rephrase, and deliver their response based on the previous answer. Take time to listen and learn from successful interviewers. Listen to their questions, hear the responses, and then listen as they rephrase the next question. Therapists will learn techniques they were unaware of.

The art of listening is an intricate part of every session. The art of listening includes hearing. Hearing is the process of perceiving sound. Listening is to heed. It is a two-step process. They call the process "Articulate listening." It simply means raising your "heed" level a few notches, and externally displaying your attentiveness to the speaker.

An aphorism calls good communication "speaking without offending, listening without defending." Good communication means somebody is talking while somebody else is listening. One is a transmitter and one is the receiver. It also applies to therapy sessions. During the opening discussion, some therapists, trying to impress their clients with their expertise, often offend. If we offend, we lose trust. We may lose trust by becoming defensive when they are talking. Practice good listening with those close to you. Articulate listening can change the client's attitude during the conversation. It could also affect your own attitude.

Anyone wanting to take the learning phase a little further, can. You can practice a little exercise with someone close to you. Establish certain ground rules before you begin. Without any interruptions, each of you will have three minutes to say something to the other person. The subject may be anything about which you want to talk. It could be feelings, politics, debts, sex, or even work. Then take the next three minutes and let her give you feedback. She must tell you what she thinks she heard you say. Next, reverse the roles, and you provide the feedback after listening to her expound on any subject. The results may surprise both of you. Are there any side benefits that may surface from this exercise? Yes, many do. It may even improve your relationship! It will also fine-tune your communication and listening skills.

During the initial interview with a client many issues are taking place. She is trying to convey her feelings, emotions and thoughts to someone whom she feels has a genuine interest. The therapist, on the other hand, has many ideas floating around in his mind. These floating ideas are called cognitive clutter. A therapist's inability to focus attention can contribute to his own mental stress, self-interest, defensiveness or strong emotion.

Understand, during any conversation we all have a desire to interject our personal garbage. For example, the word "sex" takes on a variety of meanings to those hearing the word. We automatically interject childhood, parental guidance (or lack of), experience, experiments, laws, feelings, emotions, religion, values, morals and even fantasies. That is just one word in a sentence, and it can trigger so many thoughts. It is a wonder that we can communicate when we use so many different words and have to interpret so quickly.

Nobody can communicate if they do not listen.

Therapists can do several things to help them focus their attention on the client.

- Look at the client when he is speaking.
- Turn your body toward the client.
- Listen for the meaning of the words, not just the words themselves.
- Ask questions and react responsively.
- Listen for completion.
- Remember the client can read a therapist's passivity as a sign of indifference, or a lack of interest. Articulate listening results in more understanding, commitment, and cooperation.

Once a therapist has mastered the art of listening, he can apply it to the next opening and ending discussion with his client. The application of good listening techniques may change the relationship between the therapist and client. Trust begins to build, they talk more, and the results improve drastically.

Articulate listening, if anything, will help therapists formulate responsible questions. It will help therapists interpret exactly what a client may have meant. It will also help them develop the next question or set of questions.

It is most difficult not to interject our own feelings and emotions into someone's response. When we do, we begin to develop "leading" questions based on our own garbage. We all carry around old garbage somewhere in the shadows of our mind. The garbage is negative "stuff" that we have dealt with throughout our lifetime. The *stuff* encompasses a wide range of dysfunctional rubbish we thought we had disposed of, but later discover we've put neatly into suitcases and carry with us. Our garbage occasionally surfaces when others are expressing similar difficulties. Setting out our garbage at the curb for pick up by our client's mind is not wise. Mixing our old garbage with theirs is not wise and creates more false memories.

When therapists listen to clients words and phrases they must learn to interpret meaning of words quickly, make changes and develop their next question. They must learn to accomplish this in a matter of seconds. Just as talking when someone else is talking is rude, it is rude to write while your client is responding. Fortunately, when they are in a state of hypnosis, they won't see you taking notes. Unless a therapist is a master at concurrent listening and writing, he may miss an important response crucial to the recall, or key word meaningful in developing his next question.

When a therapist listens articulately, he understands more fully the client's intent, boosting the individual's appreciation of the therapist's concern.

Much weight rests on the therapist if the court system is going to accept all evidence that hypnotically crops up during recall or regression. A client may not have excellent communication skills. The responsibility rests on the therapist to be proficient in communication. Listening takes work, but it is worth the effort. Good listening is a mark of distinction, and a true index of professionalism.

REGRESSION THERAPY

Most refer to this category of hypnosis as "age regression" because it involves returning to a previous time or age. The term regression means the reversion to an earlier mental or behavioral level. The use of regression therapy is becoming readily accepted. It has become an intricate part of Recovered Memory Therapy (RMT). Today, some therapists believe regression therapy includes the return to a previous life.   Usually, the most widely accepted term is "past-life therapy." Why is there a difference? It appears the very term "regression therapy" does not invade an individual's personal belief system and is readily becoming more acceptable. However, to categorize both "regression" and "past-life therapy" to coincide with the two schools of thought, I have separated them.   Usage is the therapist's choice if first discussed with the clients.

Age regression is a memory search of a previous age. This type of regression is limited to days, months and years. The reasons for the search vary. Commonly, in hypnosis, we use age regression to revive repressed childhood memories. Whatever the reason, triggering false memories should not be a part of the regression. As in other regressive forms, if the therapist triggers false memories, most experts believe that they may be adding new images to the individual's memory bank. (See Section on Layering)

Careful planning, advanced scripting, rehearsal, and a thorough understanding of how we, as therapists, can create false memory is critical. It is even more critical to the client. The creation or triggering of false memories is unjust, unethical and unprofessional.   Therapists owe it to their clients to protect them during any recall or regressive session.

If a therapist helps the client in any way during a regressive session, by vocalizing an irresponsible word or phrase, he may have triggered false memories. If the recalled memory doesn't come from the client, it doesn't belong to the client. Therapists must always use constraint throughout a session.

If the client struggles for a word, most therapists will help. They seem to forget that the process of recall is an extensively detailed process.   The client delves into his memory bank looking for a particular event and tries to surface that image, and to find the best words to describe the scene. Therapists have a responsibility to allow them the time to accomplish that feat.

As therapists we must realize that most individuals, in their normal conscious state, have difficulty putting any scene into words. It is not part of everyone's nature to be a great story teller. Most individuals, throughout a regular day, do not take the time to describe their work or home environments in precise detail. Why then do some therapists believe that clients can do that freely in a matter of seconds? We expect them to quickly:

-obtain a state of complete relaxation

-go back in time

-recall a particular period of their life

-select a year out of that period

-select a month

-select a day

-select an hour out of that day

-select a minute out of that hour

-select the setting, state, city, town or geographical area

-select an immediate environment within their viewing range

-describe the environment completely

-establish the event

-become emotionally involved with what they are experiencing.

-describe what they are feeling

-incorporate all the people involved

-give accurate descriptions of each person, i.e., clothes, facial features, weight, color of eyes, posture, skin color, and age.

-experience any trauma, pain or discomfort

-give each an action

-explain what role they had in the process

-and finally, we want them to describe it all **in a matter of seconds.**

That is just not realistic! Sometimes our expectations are high and our patience may be running on empty. Some therapists lack patience for successful regression. Guard against it. Become involved with the art of listening.

If a therapist asks a client in a state of hypnosis to describe where he is at a particular moment, he must allow ample time for a response. If the therapist finds that the period is the month of December and the client describes a room full of brightly colored gifts tied with beautiful ribbons, but seems to hesitate and struggle on the day, do not intervene. The automatic assumption, "Is it Christmas?" It seems like a natural response.

The interjection of the word "Christmas" creates a new connotation. He may now add a scene of Christmas to his memory bank. The people in the original scene now overlap into a Christmas setting that may or may not be true.

Other events occur in December besides Christmas -- anniversaries, birthdays, weddings and probably even the celebration of divorces. Try not to assume!

Schedule regressive sessions as the last appointment for the day, allowing extra time in the event the session lasts longer than normal. This serves two purposes. It teaches patience and allows the client to take whatever time is required to accomplish his recollection. There is no pressure to hurry because the next client is waiting.

Therapists should make each client feel he is the most important client that they have. Treat him with respect. False memories should never be a client's concern. He trusts the therapist to help him recover memories from a previous period.   That trust includes recovering those memories without tainting the images.

Clients may also involve therapists in courts of law. In today's state of awareness, it is utterly impossible to know when a particular regressive session will become the topic of a legal discussion.

PAST-LIFE THERAPY

Several years ago a therapist called me with an unusual experience. He was conducting an age regression session with a client. During the session, the client took the fetal position and appeared unresponsive for a time. In a short time she relaxed and started to speak of an event involving covered wagons, a pioneer family, the majestic beauty of mountains, and her lover. She had apparently slipped into what may be a past life. Whether the scenes and events she reported were real or unreal is not the question. The importance is that the therapist recognized the situation and could continue the session. He was open enough to understand that the human mind can accommodate just about anything.

The very thought of a previous existence produces opposition among some therapists. Most of this stems from their religious belief systems. However, past-life therapy has earned a reputation as a valuable tool in uncovering hidden notions that may be affecting an individual's current behavior. Past-life therapy, in essence, is using hypnosis to help a person on a path into what he believes is a previous life. While there, he may experience an event, place, thing or person that has an impact on his life today. That unresolved entity (usually referred to as Karma) affects their life in the present. To them, a return visit is necessary in order to move forward in their present life.

Karma may not be the only reason to visit the past. Occasionally therapists may run into clients who want to experience a previous existence for their own peace of mind.

Today, some top medical doctors and therapists are using past-life therapy successfully. The very thought of a previous life to some of those therapists may be against their personal belief system. Any top professional will never let his personal belief system interfere with therapy. To impose one's personal belief-system during a session is, in essence, a form of leading.

In any discussion of past-life therapy I usually insert a disclaimer so I am not leading anybody. My belief on the subject is personal and may be entirely different from someone else's. There is no right or wrong on the subject. Past-lives, or reincarnation, may not be real to some, but this type of therapy is very real.

Past-life therapy has been, and will be, and intricate part of therapy. I know many therapists who, because of religious beliefs, refuse to conduct past-lives therapy. That is their prerogative. If the process can enhance an individual's life, I will use it.

Past-life therapy is unique in that the design of questions is a little different. Avoidance of leading questions is very important. If therapists do not allow their clients to experience the moment, to allow their recollection to run free and explore what they are experiencing, they probably cannot confront what they believe is a previous existence. The session will be of no benefit if the therapist takes them by the hand and walks the client through the therapist's own fantasies.

In past-life therapy, no member of the legal profession will ever hear or scrutinize a therapist's line of questions, unless one of them happens to be the client. However, the results of the session are just as important to the client as if it were in a court of law. Scrutiny is the responsibility of the therapist. The script used during past-life sessions deserves a once-over by the therapist. The design of questions is important. In a past-life session, for example, a therapist should never ask a client to "describe" the clothes she is wearing. He should have some sense of time & place, and some idea of what is occurring, first.

During a past-life session, asking a client to describe how she feels is wise. Another approach is to ask what she is experiencing at a particular moment. Describing feelings and experiences is protective for both therapist and client. In a client's narration are many clues that can establish a time, place, event, person or thing. Many things can be learned by the words the client uses. Words can lay the foundation for further questions. Words can also produce a link between what the client believes to be past-life and her life today.

I once had a client who had been to several other therapists for past-life sessions. He appeared frustrated over the results. Each past-life session seemed to get to a particular existence and then everything appeared to fall apart. He was uncomfortable with the previous sessions.

I agreed to try one more time. During the regression we apparently reached that frustrating period. He described some scenes to me. I understood why the other therapists may have had some difficulty. The following is an excerpt from that session. See if you can detect anything about the young man's life.

Q: "Describe what you are experiencing right now?"

A: "It is summertime. You can smell the flowers and the freshness in the air. You can feel the warmth of the sun. I feel good and am standing outside my parent's house. It is a two-story wooden house facing the ocean. It is an old house.

I am going up the stairs into the house. My mother is in the living room. I can hear that old rocking chair. My father is somewhere else in the house."

By this time, I had an inkling of what was going on, but I needed verification.

Q: "Describe your mother?"

A: "She is a wonderful lady. Soft-spoken, loving. She has soft flowing hair. You can feel her love each time she hugs you. She is filled with love."

Have you managed to figure out anything about this young man, other than that he is very sensitive? The clues began to surface:

"You can smell the flowers and the freshness in the air."

"You can feel the warmth of the sun."

"I feel good."

"I can hear that old rocking chair."

"She is soft-spoken."

"She has soft flowing hair."

"You can feel her love."

If you figured out the young man was blind you are absolutely correct. I interpreted that fact early. Apparently, his other therapists were not listening. It isn't any wonder that the session became confusing to him. The individual had a deep compassion for the blind and wanted to know where it originated. This past-life therapy session surfaced the fact that he had been blind in a previous life. It provided the answers he needed. In addition, it provided an inner comfort.

It is not important whether therapists believe in a past-life or not. Equally unimportant is whether it is true or untrue. All personal beliefs are immaterial in this setting. The therapy should take precedence over the therapist's belief system. Advanced thinkers are using past-life therapy with huge success. If they can learn to set aside their own ideologies for the betterment of their client, other therapists can too.

The individual now understands his driving compassion to help the blind. That he now feels the priority in his life to dedicate available free time to the blind is easy to justify. He feels he was once in that same situation and not everyone was as understanding as his mother. He walked out of my office feeling more in touch with his life. He had a purpose, or at least a direction. When therapists have their clients accomplish that, they have succeeded.

Past-life therapy is serious business and should have the same respect as any therapy. Avoiding any possibility of leading during the session is extremely important. (See Section on Layering)

A close friend, trying to be unique, searched for a mode of visualized transportation to use as a method of traveling backward in time. He chose to use a passenger train. This train into the past would stop at random railroad stations during the journey into previous lives. The individual would exit the train at unscheduled stops. Once on the passenger's platform, he would look for the station name to decide where he was and tell the therapist the name of the town. Does this script sound unique? Is it really?

This type of induction is perfectly acceptable, if the therapist knows for sure that the client's trip into a previous existence occurred since the discovery of the railroad, approximately one hundred and sixty-five years ago. However, the therapist may be placing limits on previous existence by mere mention of a railroad. The mention of a railroad is leading and could add or create a false memory.

Using this clever scenario is also perfectly permissible if the client was not blind, or even illiterate in her previous life. In either case, she could not possibly read the station sign, or even find it. It could be feasible if her prior existence had been spent in a railroad town. What if she had a tremendous fear of trains? I would never criticize anyone for being unique. For some, uniqueness is important. Unique or not, scrutiny of scripts is always important. Remember, if the therapist limits the client in any manner including wording, setting, impatience, phraseology, script, music, interruption or simply by not listening, he could be leading and creating false memories.

TRANSFERENCE AND FALSE MEMORIES

Transference is the act or process of transferring. When we add the word "feelings" into that definition it begins to take on a different connotation. In essence, the client begins to have feelings about the therapist as a person.

The reasons for transference are many. The client, during early sessions, began a process of trust. The process gradually incorporates other emotions and feelings. She feels a comfort and closeness for the therapist. Sometimes, it does not stop there. In the client's eye, the therapist is almost "Godlike." To some therapists, the very thought of a client transferring feelings toward them seems totally ridiculous. We must remember, we as therapists are also dealing with our own inadequacies. It is those inadequacies that get in the way. A few therapists are narrow minded enough to believe that transference could not take place. They may rationalize with, "My client is a beautiful person, and what would they want with me?" They may also use this thought provoking rationale: "She is young and I am old enough to be her father."

A certain amount of transference takes place with many people throughout a normal day. Place anyone in a situation of comfort, closeness and trust and the early stages of transference occur. We have all experienced instances of closeness and comfort with complete strangers. In those instances, we were probably aware of our feelings. What would happen if were not aware of the process of transference and felt a strong attachment to that person? Both therapist and client are subject to that sometimes occurring.

Feelings of comfort and closeness surface in a client because the therapist appears genuinely to care. She believes that no one else in her life cares. The therapist also listens intently to what she has to say. Gradually, deeper feelings emerge. A professional therapist has to curtail those deeper feelings early with kindness, sensitivity, and professionalism. If they do not, distrust, instability in future relationships, and even hate may result.

A link exists between transference and triggering false memories. If the therapist inappropriately triggers a false memory, the client may believe that the therapist has uncovered an unresolved situation or devastation in her life. By falsely triggering that memory, she may become dependent on the therapist, who seemingly has freed her from a horrible trauma. She may begin to look to the therapist as her "savior." As that misinterpretation begins to form, transference has already started. Transference may also occur if the trauma is revealed without a therapist leading.

Another side of the coin exists. Some therapists become opportunists. They enjoy it when the compliments received from clients stroke their egos. In a subsequent session, the therapist may embellish the false memories, knowingly or unknowingly, just to receive more strokes.

The therapist may not even be aware of the full impact of his impoverished pride. The consequences of triggering false memories or embellishment can be catastrophic to everyone concerned. Transference readily occurs as the new layers of false memories take form. The client, through whatever process, may begin to see how blaming her difficulties on someone else is easy. She is grateful to the therapist for making everything clear and clean. In actuality, the therapist has dirtied the air and subsequently a law suit may follow. Secondly, his foolish pride has paved the way for utter confusion.

Prevention of a negative scenario is preventable with a little knowledge. Therapists should be aware. They should be professional enough to understand fully that transference takes place unexpectedly and in a variety of forms. Therapists must tune into words spoken by their clients, and listen to the feelings and emotions behind each word. They should avoid embellishing any thought, scene or description, during any recall session. Therapists must make every effort to guarantee that their client's words belongs to them. Keep your private thoughts private.

"Only God is in a position to look down on anyone."
                                          -Sarah Brown

"Some people change their ways when they see the light; others when they feel the heat."

Caroline Schoeder

CHAPTER FIVE

LEGALITIES

Is there a lighter side to false memories? There is, if you consider the latest "question and answer" jokes centered on therapists.

Question: "What did the judge say to the therapist dressed in a three-piece business suit?"

Answer: "Would the defendant please rise?"

If therapists are not going to take seriously the business of providing leading questions, they may very well hear those words.

Too many therapists ignore the consequences of providing "leading" questions. Pick up any daily newspaper or watch the evening news on television. Hundreds of individuals may be in jail for crimes they never committed.

Individuals claiming abuse and their families are being scarred for life. Restoring control to the victim is a widely recognized part of therapy. Often, therapists will lead their clients to believe that bringing suppressed memories to the surface will remove all damaging psychological symptoms. Frequently that assumption is true. However, with the interjection of leading questions during regression, the opposite happens. Their situation usually worsens and clients experience a sad separation from their loved ones. Thousands of lives enter chaos and mass hysteria because of therapists leading questions that trigger false memories.

Some individuals arrive at a therapist's office with preconceived suspicions of childhood sexual abuse. They are looking for the authority figure who might support them in their search. The suspicions may surface at anytime. A 44-year-old Long Island, New York woman, a registered nurse, sued a priest for sexually abusing her at the age of fifteen. She had watched "The Home Show" the day before, with guest star Margaux Hemingway, who discussed sexual abuse and eating disorders. The next morning the NY woman recalled her own sexual abuse and took action to sue. From a therapeutic perspective, such lawsuits could prove valuable in helping victims retake or reassert control of their lives. Simultaneously, the court systems are requiring standards of proof before allowing suits based on recovered memories to be filed.

"The therapists who are doing this (Recovered Memory Therapy) are a new kind of sexual predator. Without ever touching their victims, they move them as close as you can possibly get to experience rape and brutalization...And they get paid by the hour for doing it."

Richard Ofshe, Ph.D.

Do therapists inform their client's of the risks and dangers of slight suggestion? If they warn them up front, what they can expect to uncover? Such a warning may begin the process of creation of false memories.

Because therapists have not taken the time for training, or appear blasé about the interjection of leading questions, their actions have triggered the largest controversy within the psychological arena and court system today. The controversy stems from childhood sexual abuse based on recovered memories. Untrained therapists are leading clients to believe in abuse that never happened. They are advising their patients that their symptoms are characteristic of childhood abuse, even when the client denies the abuse. When the trusted therapist speaks of characteristic traits the client takes heed and turns it into a "high-probability." The result: overcrowded court rooms, broken families, rich attorneys, and trauma beyond your wildest imagination. In addition, they are establishing precedents in the United States for civil action against therapists who surface false memories.

Relating the triggering of false memories to a small child who is constantly asking his mother for some candy is not difficult. If the child asks for the candy enough times, he may get what he asks for. He may ask for the candy in a variety of ways, until eventually his mother gives in. The therapist, asking for something enough times, will eventually get it. This drill fringes upon unethical and inappropriate practice.

The sad commentary of the controversy is that many therapists are being indicted. Whether or not he wishes for any involvement in a court battle, he often becomes a central figure. The action of a few will draw all therapists into the arena. Each of us will confront the public, friends, family, office staff and local reporters. We will spend valuable time trying to defend the profession. It will take each of us individually to suppress the controversy and clean up the profession. The first step toward better understanding of the problem is an awareness of the situation. Many books are available on the subject. Several organizations such as the False Memory Syndrome Foundation (FMSF) are now available to provide training and to teach the therapists how to protect his client and his derriere.

A nationwide alert and awareness are surfacing on the problem of child-sexual abuse, and it should be. Childhood sexual abuse is a real and serious crime. According to the National Committee to Prevent Child Abuse, more than two hundred thousand reported cases occur each year. The cases are serious enough to warrant serious investigation. The crux of this dilemma is that there are thousands of cases no one will report. And today, more people are accusing, suing and judging based on testimony of abuse that may be more "make-believe" than memory.

The laws are changing. Today, every state in the Union is developing laws to protect children against sexual abuse. They are also changing laws governing when victims may sue therapists over reports of repressed memories of abuse. The numbers of suits are increasing daily. Many suits have stemmed from the therapists requests that their clients confront their abusers. Therapists have a unique relationship with their clients based on honor and trust. A trusted therapist can influence what an individual reports, including memories of abuse. If they violate that circumstance, they have created another abuse.

Most therapists are caring, loving and ethical people who sincerely want to help. If this is true, and it is, then where did all the misunderstandings begin? Probably the most publicized case was Eileen Franklin-Lipsker's recovered memory of the murder of a childhood girlfriend. Her recall of the event led to the arrest of her own father. Consequently, the case went to trial and a conviction followed. That trial and subsequent publicity have triggered hundreds of cases throughout the nation. Next, the news media locked on the much publicized child sexual abuse trial of the North Carolina Little Rascals Day Care Center owners. Others followed, including accusations of sexual abuse of Cardinal Joseph Bernardin, one of the most respected leaders within the Catholic church. The recovered memory was something that occurred seventeen years ago. His accuser, Steven Cook, later retracted his suit. The reason affected the field of hypnosis. Mr. Cook said his memories were unreliable because the therapist who conducted the session was unqualified to practice hypnosis. Later, the news media quoted Cardinal Bernardin as saying, "My life will never be the same because of this man." The impact of accusations based on false memories is devastating.

A day care worker at the Wee Care Day Nursery in Maplewood, New Jersey, received a conviction for molesting children. In 1993, an appeals court overturned her conviction. An individual's right to a fair trial was the basis of the appeal. The appeal judges based their decision on the "leading" manner in which the children underwent questioning before the trial. This trial precipitated many questions. One question was asked during a discussion with other therapists: Are there therapists so eager for publicity that they are willing to endanger the lives of so many people? On the other hand, we must seriously consider the impact of true abuse on children. In an effort to hurriedly get repressed memories surfaced, and possibly into the court system, therapists may not be bringing a truly guilty person to justice.

The American Medical Association (AMA) recently

passed a resolution warning doctors that hypnosis and other types of memory enhancement techniques may produce stories of events that never really occurred. The AMA made the following statement June 16, 1994, in their Report of the Council of Scientific Affairs, CSA Report 5-A-94 titled *Memories of Childhood Abuse.* "The AMA considers recovered memories of childhood sexual abuse to be of uncertain authenticity, which should be subject to external verification." The idea of proving that a recovered memory, (with or without hypnosis) is false, is just as difficult as proving a conscious recalled memory is true.

The AMA Report also addressed legal concerns. "To some extent, current concerns about repressed memories can be traced to the lawsuits filed by accusers, particularly those filed against parents. Numerous such lawsuits have been filed by accusers, and it is of course difficult to disprove accusations regarding events that are alleged to have taken place many years or even decades earlier. Over the past few years, a number of states have adopted laws that have affected such litigation. Illinois, for example, has just extended the time allowed in which to file a suit; previously lawsuits could not be filed after the accuser had attained the age of 30. On the other hand, California has recently adopted laws under which a plaintiff cannot prevail in the absence of evidence beyond the recovered memories."

Some of the individuals and families affected by accusations of false memories have united to form the False Memory Syndrome Foundation, based in Philadelphia, Pennsylvania.

We all know and accept that the human brain is a unique, powerful, yet mystical organ. We know that an individual's mind can block some horrid, painful events, forever. It is a way of protecting us from reexperiencing that suffering, agonizing pain. We also realize that researchers will spend the next two thousand years before they fully understand all the workings of our mind, its memory bank and why it protects us.

A therapist's practice is nothing more than a distinct reflection of who he is. Some people have haunting and horrid memories. The exploitation of those memories by noted therapists are resulting in serious civil charges. Those charges have brought some scum to the surface, and rightfully so. Childhood abuse is serious, and complete eradication should be everyone's objective. Leading someone on a path of false memories is just as serious and should also face eradication.

Therapists who lead should have their licenses revoked. Leading is a power issue, wherein the therapist feels a need to have control over someone. Besides the unprofessional conduct of leading, national studies report that 9% of medical doctors, psychiatrists, psychologists, therapists and counselors admit to personal sexual misconduct. A therapy setting does not always lend itself to a third party in the room during a session. However, that does not mean that therapists cannot, and should not, protect both themselves and the client from possible irregularities. Electronic technology has paralleled the demand for protection. Just as the subtle video camera can capture the robbers of the all-night convenience store, it can also protect both the therapist and the client.

FORENSIC REGRESSION

During the lifetime of a therapist, an agency of the law may ask him to consider conducting a regression of an individual. Some agencies do not realize that forensic hypnosis is a specialized field. If a therapist does not have the proper training in forensic hypnosis, he is better off to refer law enforcement officials to someone else. Most individuals do not follow that advice. It titillates the ego to be asked to be part of an investigation. The inquiry alone provides the necessary strokes. Our ego wants to be the *Perry Mason* of the day and have a major role in solving the case. In reality, it may be the ego that gets in the way, as it does in so many other situations. If someone qualified in forensic hypnosis cannot be found a therapist properly trained in hypnosis regression could feasibly conduct the regression if he meets certain criteria.

Before any therapist accepts the task, he should ask himself if he can handle it properly. Before any therapist embarks on such a venture it is wise to be aware of several important objectives relating to forensic regressions.

(1) The very case requiring a therapist's services may be solely dependent on the specifics obtained and the phrasing of the questions.

(2) The therapist should understand the importance of wording.

(3) The therapist should always ask questions of those handling the investigation.

(4) Everyone should be clear on the objective of the regression.

(5) What is the focus of the regression? Is it for informational purposes only? Are there specifics that need to surface?

(6) Develop your line of questioning in advance. A careless therapist's line of questioning could prove damaging, setting an expensive investigation back for days, months or even years. It could also set a guilty man free or send an innocent man to prison.

In some situations, the regression may be better off with less detailed information about the case before the induction. In those specific instances, less information will reduce their chances of interjecting any leading questions. With less information, the use of well developed questions could avoid tainting or contaminating any response of the client. Investigators should understand the details regarding the use of hypnosis. They should also understand how, in some circumstances, the less information the regressor has increases the chances of getting accurate responses. The therapist's involvement should be in alignment with the objective of the regression, and not as an investigator. It is important therapists understand the difference.

In other circumstances, the therapist may be better off reviewing the documented history of the case, gaining as much information as he can before developing the line of questions. That contradicts the previous paragraph, however a reason does exist for this inconsistency: The objective of the case. What type of information will the regression uncover? Is there a possibility of an admission of guilt? Is there an alternative list of questions to handle newly uncovered information? Has the list undergone scrutiny by both the defense and prosecution? If the developed list has not received approval before the regression, any information revealed by the individual may be futile. If the judge does allow the information, the office that introduces the information has an obligation to verify each point.

How do we know whether essential information will hinder or aid the line of questioning during any regression? The objective of the case will provide the information needed for the decision. For example, if the prosecution is looking only for leads and other information related to the case, then detailed information concerning the case could be beneficial.

If they are looking for the individual's involvement, the therapist may have to consider less information. Does law enforcement suspect the individual's involvement in a brutal attack of another individual? If they do, the weapon used might be crucial. In a regressive state, the suspect may reveal critical information that only the police and the attackers know. The fewer details the therapist knows of the weapon the less chance he has of leading the suspect in regression. To seek less information or more information may appear to be a difficult decision. Once law enforcement establishes the objectives, the decision is less difficult. In the preliminary interview with the authorities, the therapist should always explain his role in the process. The therapist should explain how knowledge of the regression objective is important. He should also explain why he should have more or fewer details concerning the case. If the therapist expresses his concern to surface information without contamination, his credibility is strengthened and participation on other regressions is highly probable.

Everyone involved with various aspects of a case can be subject to cross examination and even to criminal charges if it is found that they interfered with the process. Recently, charges were filed in Los Angeles against a Korean interpreter who embellished a victim's testimony during a rape case. The interpreter, angered by the suspect's acts of violence, altered and omitted portions of the testimony of the victim. The woman accused her ex-boyfriend of kidnapping, sexually assaulting and beating her. Her story didn't appear strong enough to the interpreter, who feared she might lose the case. Embellishment seemed a natural thing to do.

Is there any difference between falsely embellishing the testimony of a victim or creating false memories by "leading" the client? The process is different. However, some leading therapists believe the insertion of "leading questions" should carry the same seriousness and scrutiny as an embellished testimony. "Leading questions" would then face a possible loss to antiquity, never to enter a forensic hypnosis session again.

From the information the investigators provide, the therapist should develop a list of questions. All parties concerned should review these before the actual regression. Verifying with all parties associated with the case that the questions are not in any way leading is necessary for the courts. Once the list appears to satisfy everyone, the regression can continue.

Whether the investigators require it or not, the session should be conspicuously video taped. Always include a backup audio recording of the session. The therapist must be careful not to alter any questions. However, he must be flexible enough to develop another question if the need arises based on the client's answers. Forensic regression is time consuming, critical, valuable, and informative. Forensic hypnosis training, available through many reputable organizations would be advantageous for all therapists.

Modern law enforcement agencies are now recruiting or training staff members in forensic regression. However, the possibility of obtaining outside services always exists. Prepare yourself for the inevitable.

DEPARTMENT OF JUSTICE

Excluding the views of the highest law enforcement agency in the United States, when writing about hypnosis and memory recall, would be inappropriate. Memory recall is the process that supports all of the testimony spoken in courts across the nation. Every individual on every witness stand throughout the world is using some form of memory recall. How accurate and complete is their recall of events? Even the Attorney General's Office of the Department of Justice relies on hypnosis as a tool to obtain some information. Exactly what position does the Department of Justice take regarding hypnosis, the triggering of false memories, and leading questions?

The Department of Justice Manual outlines strict guidance regarding the use of hypnosis. They realize the use of hypnosis is important and can aid in the investigative process. In the United States Attorneys' Manual, page 22, it clearly states their objectives. **"Witnesses to crimes have been able to recall certain facets of the crime while in a hypnotic state that they could not remember in the normal state."**

The guidance to their employees takes on an overtone of caution that probably is traceable to the public, and maybe voices the court's objection. **"Hypnosis, however, is subject to serious objections and should be used only on rare occasions. The information obtained from a person while in a hypnotic trance cannot be assumed to be accurate."**

The difference begins, between those in the field of hypnosis and those in the Justice Department, when it is suggested the hypnosis recall was inaccurate. The advice in their manual should state, **"All conscious recall of events cannot be assumed to be accurate. However, memory recall through the application of hypnosis, properly induced and properly questioned, can provide the most accurate information available."**

We are constantly storing information in the mind. Surfacing the information with hypnosis does require an adept therapist. The therapist must possess the same concerns as the investigators in obtaining accuracy. With passively developed questions, accurate information is possible through hypnosis recall. Naturally, any information obtained with hypnosis should undergo verification for accuracy and corroboration.

Their manual also advises staff to take every precaution, just as all therapists should do during every recall session. Research associated with recall finds that information obtained from a hypnosis state is reliable. Individuals in a hypnotic state can recall sound, detailed information not normally available to them in a conscious state. The differences rest in the line of questioning used to obtain the information. It is that simple.

Once the information is obtained through hypnotically refreshed memory, is that evidence admissible in a trial? The question is open in many jurisdictions. The manual addresses admissibility. **"In those jurisdictions in which the question is unsettled, a foundation concerning the reliability of hypnosis is necessary."**

Many cases have surfaced where information obtained through hypnosis is inadmissible in court. Certain court systems, jurisdictions and/or regions are more receptive in the use of hypnosis. **"In jurisdictions where such evidence is clearly admissible, there is no foundation concerning the nature and effects of hypnosis."**

The manual lengthens their protection by offering some definition. **"The courts that permit the use of hypnotically induced testimony by prosecution witnesses have held that the fact of the hypnosis affects only the credibility of the witness and not the witness's competence or the admissibility of his or her testimony."**

They specifically address cases involving the use of hypnosis and its acceptance in the manual. In a case *United States versus Adams*, the Ninth Circuit Court upheld the admissibility of hypnotically refreshed testimony but the court expressed concern. **"Investigatory use of hypnosis on persons who may later be called upon to testify in court carries a dangerous potential for abuse. Great care must be exercised to insure that statements after hypnosis are the production of the subject's own recollection, rather than of recall *tainted* by suggestions received while under hypnosis."**

RECORDING

In that same case, the courts said, **"At a minimum, complete stenographic records of interviews of hypnotized persons who later testify should be maintained. Only if the judge, jury, and the opponent know who was present, questions that were asked, and the witness's responses can the matter be dealt with effectively. An audio or video recording of the interview would be helpful."**

Recordings and backup material become the mainstay of pretrial hypnosis. No one can overemphasize the importance of such records. The generally accepted admissibility of testimony refreshed or unlocked by pretrial hypnosis should always have proper documentation.

CONSENT

The manual also addresses the need of hypnosis and consent. **"Hypnosis of a witness should not be employed unless there is a clear need for additional information, and it appears that hypnosis can be useful in aiding the witness to recall such information. A witness should never be hypnotized unless the witness gives consent,** preferably in writing, and the witness should always be given an explanation of the nature of hypnosis before being hypnotized."

WHO SHOULD PERFORM HYPNOSIS?

Does the Department of Justice eliminate therapists from inducing hypnosis on any individual involved in their cases? No. However, it offers a recommendation to the members of their Department. **"Only a person trained in the art of hypnosis should be allowed to hypnotize a witness. During the interrogation, leading questions should be avoided to insure against the possibility of suggestion to the subject."**

Always prove the legitimacy of your questions during any recall session with recordings. The Justice Department is aware how important recordings are to any case. All therapists should be aware too. **"Interrogation made when the witness is subject to hypnosis should be videotaped whenever possible. In those cases where videotaping the interview is impossible, a transcript should be prepared in addition to any sound recording. Where the interview is videotaped, the tape need not be transcribed unless it is necessary in subsequent legal proceedings to provide a transcript. However, where a videotape is made but the interview is not transcribed, a copy of the videotape should be made to guard against the loss of or damage to the original tape."**

SUPREME COURT RULING

On June 22, 1987, the Supreme Court found unconstitutional as a violation of the Fifth, Sixth, and

Fourteenth Amendments, an Arkansas rule excluding a criminal defendant's hypnotically refreshed testimony. While the Supreme Court was **'not prepared to endorse without qualifications the use of hypnosis as an investigative tool,'** it did conclude that a state's legitimate interest in excluding unreliable evidence **'does not justify a mandatory exclusionary rule barring a defendant's hypnotically refreshed testimony because such testimony could be reliable in an individual case.'** In the 1987 decision, the court went on to suggest that the states establish guidelines to help the trial courts evaluate the validity of hypnotically enhanced testimony in any case. The procedures would aid in assessing the accuracy of testimony refreshed hypnotically. They also suggested the procedures include the use of trained personnel, and videotaping and recording the hypnotic sessions.

It is interesting that the manual of the Justice Department also states that, **"If a witness has been hypnotized prior to trial, this fact should be disclosed in court and the defendant should be given such information. In many cases, of course, the government will be required to produce the witness's prior statements."** It is a form of protection for all concerned. Disclosure of all the facts and information surrounding the case is available to everyone. The information includes the scripts developed by the therapist.

HYPNOSIS EXPERTS EXPECTED TO TESTIFY

The manual concludes with a suggestion of protection for the Department. **"The prosecution should be prepared to put on the stand an expert on hypnosis who can explain to the jury the nature of hypnosis and how it works in the**

**interrogation process in order to dispel from the jurors'
minds any misconceptions and doubts they may have
concerning hypnosis."**

Therapists know that the process of dispelling the
juror's doubts, myths, and notions concerning hypnosis is
essential. Members of the court, jury, attorneys, defendant
and the accused are not exempt from those same explanations
and information. The therapist's efforts may not end there.
He should prepare to explain his line of questioning. He may
need to defend wording, phraseology, knowledge and script.
A therapist may have to testify. The skeptics are waiting.

"To do injustice is more disgraceful than to suffer it."
-Plato

"The only tyrant I accept in this world
is still the small voice within me."

Mahatma Gandhi

CHAPTER SIX

ETHICS

Do therapists always live up to the lofty standards
expected of them? Some do not, and they eventually make the
headlines of the local newspapers and television news. Like
everyone else, therapists are human. Most therapists want to
be ethical and will do everything in their power to avoid
triggering false memories. However, without the proper
training or knowledge they may be putting too much trust in
their personal experiences. If they are, a strong possibility
exists they may be deceiving themselves. They may be
allowing their own ambition to interfere with a successful
recall session. Maybe they are simply not aware of their use
of leading words or phrases, setting the stage for mass
confusion. Without the awareness and knowledge of

"leading," their own passion to be exceptional may cloud their objectivity.

Today, systems are in place to provide checks and balances. Therapists should take the steps necessary to provide a critique of their clinical techniques and practices. If they don't, they need not worry about them. They will provide the service in the courtrooms across America, and the attorneys and judges will provide the necessary scrutiny. If every therapist has done his or her homework, the information obtained during a recall session can withstand cross examination by any of the skeptics. Every client takes his therapist on a unique and absorbing journey through the jungles of the mind, through the caverns of the soul. Let us hold up our lanterns to illuminate the undisguised truth, to be plain and just and ethical in our dealings all along the way.

"If you think you did something that may be unethical, it may already be too late."

Every time we complete a journey another one awaits. I hope you have enjoyed the trip.

BIBLIOGRAPHY

Brussel, James A., MD   1969
The Layman's Guide to Psychiatry
New York: Barnes & Noble, Inc.

Coble, Yank D., Jr., MD, Chair   1994
AMA Report of the Council on Scientific Affairs
Chicago, IL: Report

Fear, Richard A.,   1978
The Evaluation Interview
New York: McGraw Hill, Inc.

Kagan, Jerome & Havemann, Ernest   1972
Psychology: An Introduction
New York: Harcourt Brace Jovanovich, Inc.

Kroger, William S., MD, Fezler, William D., Ph.D.   1976
*Hypnosis and Behavior Modification: Imagery
            Conditioning*
Philadelphia: J. B. Lippincott Company

Ofshe, Richard, Ph.D.   1994
*How Things Go Wrong in Recovered Memory
            Therapy*
Philadelphia, PA: False Memory Syndrome
            Foundation Newsletter

Staff, Readers Digest,   1990
ABC's of the Human Mind
Pleasantville, NY: Reader Digest Books

Wade, Carol & Tavris, Carol   1990
Psychology, Second Edition
New York: Harper & Row

Order Form

For additional copies of *Hypnosis and False Memories: How False Memories Are Created* you may contact your local bookseller or use this handy coupon:

Send to:
Ziotech International
Attn. Ordering Dept.
617 High Street
Freeport, PA 16229-1223

Please send me an additional copy of *Hypnosis and False Memories: How False Memories Are Created.* (I am enclosing $12.95 plus $1.50 for shipping and handling.) Send check or money order - no cash or C.O.D.'s please.

Name: _____

Address: _____

City_____ State____Zip _____

Please allow three weeks for delivery

Please add my name to the Ziotech International mailing list so I may receive announcements of upcoming publications.

INDEX

The Author

Ronald L. Stephens began his studies in hypnosis in the early 70's with Dr. William Kroger, MD, of UCLA, a pioneer in Clinical Hypnosis. Later, he opened the Intermountain Hypnosis Center in Salt Lake City, Utah, for behavior modification and classes on self hypnosis.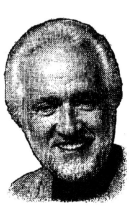

Through the years, Mr. Stephens also pursued a career in another arena. During his own pursuit of self attainment, he developed an interest in the philosophy of metaphysics and its impact of mind, body and spirit. He pursued his interest and obtained his Doctorate in Metaphysical Science in 1988. Today, he is gaining national recognition for his contribution in the metaphysical arena as an ordained Minister affiliated with the National Metaphysics Institute and the International New Thought Alliance.

His involvement in the business community has earned him the privilege of being selected as an honored member of Who's Who in US Executives.

During his years of private practice he developed a keen interest in the correlation of false memories and individuals in a highly suggestible state of hypnosis. News spread of Dr. Stephens knowledge on the subject. He became a dependable source for fellow therapists, police agencies, researchers and teachers in search of guidance. Their encouragement became the driving force behind this book. As he shares his perceptions in this book, the author believes this work will enlighten many on the creation of false memories in a therapy environment.

Recently, speaking to a group of therapists, Dr. Stephens said, "Therapists have a responsibility to understand how much influence they have in the creation of false memories. They also have a responsibility to protect their clients and rid society of potentially damaging false memories that inept therapy can possibly create. A therapists' search for excellence must not end with this book. This book is only a beginning."